THE SALON BIZ
Tips for Success

GERI MATAYA

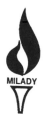

Milady Publishing Company
(A Division of Delmar Publishers Inc.)
3 Columbia Circle, Box 15-015
Albany, New York 12212

NOTICE TO THE READER

Editor: Catherine Frangie
Developmental Editor: Joseph Miranda
Editorial Assistant: Denise Brienza
Editing Supervisor: Marlene McHugh Pratt
Project Editor: Pamela Fuller
Production Manager: John Mickelbank
Illustrator: Cathy Harr, Harr Productions

Copyright © 1992
Milady Publishing Company
(A Division of Delmar Publishers Inc.)

Printed in the United States of America

10 9 8 7 6 5 4 3 2

Library of Congress Cataloging-in-Publication Data
Mataya, Geri
    The salon biz: tips for success / by Geri Mataya.
      p.   cm.
    ISBN 1–56253–048–8
    1. Beauty shops—Management. I. Title.
TT965.M38   1992
646.7'2'068—dc20   92-9492
                                                  CIP

CONTENTS

DEDICATION

This book is lovingly dedicated to my husband Ron for always being there to support my efforts, to my children Mark and Scott for their understanding and ability to pick up the ball when I wasn't able to be there due to my many involvements outside our home, to my mom for her encouragement and the consistent demonstration of love, devotion, and work ethics that she gave me.

And finally to the memory of Mr. Felix, owner of Maison Felix Beauty School, who believed in me enough to give me a scholarship, which began my career in cosmetology.

ACKNOWLEDGMENTS

When I think of the number of people who inspired and enriched my life, it is mind boggling. I am so grateful to all the wonderful people who helped make a difference in my life. I would like to thank my dear friends in the business, especially:

Andoni Lizardy and Walter Brown, authors of *Achieving Your Heart's Desire*s, who taught me how to set and carry out my goals and also for allowing me to use some of their information on goal setting;

John and Maryanne McCormick, owners of Visible Changes, Houston, Texas, for helping and supporting me when times were tough;

Izear Winfrey, my true friend and employee, for his help, moral support, and dependability, and for always being there when I needed someone to talk to;

To all of my friends at Intercoiffure and NCA;

To all of my staff members past and present, who have taught me how to be a leader, for motivating and inspiring me, for sometimes forcing me to make decisions that were uncomfortable, and for making me a stronger person;

To all of the wonderful people I've met in my career — employers, clients, stylists, manufacturers, editors, show organizers, and salon owners — whose guiding words, enthusiasm, and love of the industry have given me the inspiration to succeed.

FROM THE AUTHOR

It seems that the longer I'm in the beauty business, the more I grow to love it. This business has been so good to me professionally as well as personally!

Cosmetology has given me the opportunity to grow in all aspects of my life. It has allowed me to travel, share ideas, and meet thousands of people all over the world. I know firsthand that this is a spectacular profession that has so much to offer, and I welcomed the chance to share my knowledge and experience with others in the industry.

I guess this was one of the reasons I decided to write this book — so that people could see all of the valuable things that are available to our industry — over and above "just cutting hair."

I hope you will use this book for inspiration, motivation, and excitement so you too can become whoever and whatever you want to be. Set your goals, create your image, and focus your mind on achieving your creation. I know that you will be wildly successful!

MANAGEMENT

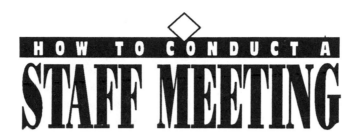

HOW TO CONDUCT A
STAFF MEETING

Monthly staff meetings are very important for a smooth-running salon. They keep the staff informed about what is going on in management and give them a chance to discuss their concerns and ideas. Not to be used as a gripe session, they should be positive and productive. Here are some guidelines to follow.

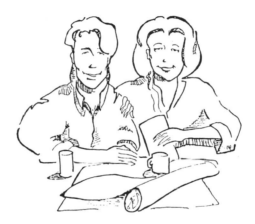

PREPARATION CHECKLIST

1. At least one week ahead of time, prepare a letter stating the date, time, and place of the meeting, and display it on your bulletin board, or send a copy to each staff member. Include the topics for discussion, allowing everyone to be prepared to ask or answer questions. Breakfast meetings work well because people are fresh in the morning. Suggestions: You might want to serve coffee, juice and/or snacks if it is very early. Feed the body as well as the mind, and your staff will love you.
2. Have a time frame in mind for each discussion topic and stick to your agenda.
3. Make sure any written information you wish to distribute is available before the meeting.
4. Make it a habit to begin your meetings on time. Insist that everyone be punctual.

THE GAME PLAN

Prior to the meeting, it's a good idea to have a motivational tape playing while people are gathering together. This will help them get "psyched up."

Appoint a secretary to record everything that is discussed during the meeting. Begin by having someone read the minutes from the last session, then briefly follow up on any assignments you might have given. Lavishly praise those who have responded positively, but take care of any negative issues privately whenever possible.

Allow your staff to get involved with the business by giving you their ideas and suggestions for sales and service improvements. Get the opinions of the quiet members, and be sure to retain control over the talkers. There are always a few individuals who dominate every group. Make sure they don't monopolize your time. Have a roll call at every meeting, and have staff members account for the amount of time they spend promoting themselves and building their clienteles. We are in the sales business, and it is important for each person to be responsible for increasing his/her book. If you have someone who is extremely busy, have that person help the others by explaining how to increase client base and how certain services keep the client coming back.

Next, discuss how you can improve your customer service. This is the most important aspect of your business. One suggestion is to have your customers fill out a questionnaire on the quality of service given by each of your employees. This information can help your salon business continually grow.

Talk about new ideas to promote business and staff members. Consider the cleanliness of the salon, and discuss ways of improving its appearance. Encourage your employees to get involved in outside activities. A well-rounded employee is a happier and more interesting person and a better worker. Help employees set goals and discover new ways of attaining them. If they are uncomfortable with selling, role-play with them. Talk about teamwork and how they can work together to get the job done. Put more than one person on a project so they can learn from one another.

End your meeting on a positive note. Help your people to get excited about their careers!

TIPS

- *Always keep your meeting positive!*
- *Don't let personal feelings cause you to be angry or negative.*
- *Don't let personalities run your meeting.*
- *Don't beat a subject into the ground. Allow yourself enough time to deal with it, and then move on to the next thing.*
- *Keep track of who is doing what, and make sure that jobs are completed.*
- *Don't make promises you can't deliver or agree to something you are unable or unwilling to do.*
- *NEVER embarrass an employee in front of the staff, but ALWAYS be willing to praise and encourage your people in front of anyone and everyone! They will respond as positively as they are treated!*
- *HAVE A GREAT STAFF MEETING!!!*

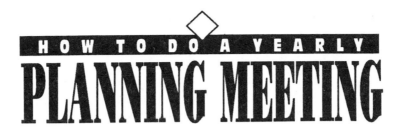

HOW TO DO A YEARLY PLANNING MEETING

With a new year comes a chance to plan ways of making the coming twelve months more prosperous and enjoyable for everyone on your staff. It's also a great opportunity to allow the creativity of your people to flow and for everyone to get involved and really feel like part of the team.

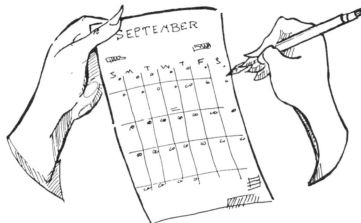

PREPARATION CHECKLIST

1. Choose a time and place for your meeting. It's great to rent a room for the day, because it gets you into a new environment and away from the salon. Have the hotel provide meals and snacks so you aren't interrupted. Make it a pleasant and productive atmosphere.

2. Have an agenda prepared beforehand. You might ask for ideas about possible topics at your December staff meeting in order to get input from your staff members. Remember to include salon and staff goals, incentives, and bonuses.

3. Organize all of your information concerning ideas and figures from the previous year. This will include such subjects as advertising, promotions, photo sessions, mailings, salon prices, hours, training, shows, etc. Know which thoughts worked and which didn't so you can incorporate the successful ones into your new plan.

4. Bring taping or video equipment to record your meeting so your ideas do not get lost or misinterpreted.

5. Have butcher paper and markers and/or plenty of pens and paper to keep track of everything.

6. Make sure everyone comes prepared to contribute. Tell them to bring their brains wrapped in their best ideas.

THE GAME PLAN

Begin by talking to your people about your salon and its goals. Discuss your business philosophy (clients — without them there is no business; corporation — includes everyone as a whole; and, finally, the individual) and how you view yourself in the marketplace. Tell them why it is important for them to be involved in this decision-making process.

After everyone is involved, go through a worksheet for each month and determine what must be done daily to achieve the month's goals. Assign jobs to specific people with completion dates. Go over the corporate structure, how each individual fits into it, and where he can go. Discuss strengths and needs and how you can improve every aspect of your business. Encourage everyone to participate, but have a timeframe for each subject and do your best to stay with it so you don't lose control of your meeting.

Now you're ready to plan. Make up a large calendar for the year. Suggestion: Butcher paper can be hung on the walls; you can sketch your calendar, and everyone can see. Go through each month and set dates for promotions, photo shoots, salon activities, training seminars, meetings, assignments, etc.

End on a positive note with a summary of the ideas of the day. Leave everyone with excitement and anticipation for the coming year.

TIPS

- *Your monthly worksheets are a roadmap for the coming year. Though they can be altered if necessary, try to follow them as closely as you can, for this allows you to plan and budget your time and money for a successful marketing strategy.*
- *Don't be afraid to go to friends in other businesses for ideas on planning and marketing.*
- *Do goal graphs for each staff member in all aspects of life — personal, professional, social, etc. Help staff members visualize their goals, which will in turn help them to achieve those goals.*
- *Do a lot of brainstorming, and don't necessarily dismiss what seems at first like a crazy idea. Sometimes they can develop into some of your best promotions.*
- *Be aware of what a great opportunity this meeting is for your staff relationships and for your business. Use your time wisely and creatively.*
- *REMEMBER, NO BUSINESS CAN SUCCEED UNLESS YOU KNOW WHERE YOU ARE GOING AND HOW YOU ARE GOING TO GET THERE!*

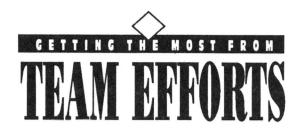

GETTING THE MOST FROM
TEAM EFFORTS

Athletics are a great way to measure teamwork. Without the work of everyone on the football field, you can't win a game. This is also true in your organization.

PREPARATION CHECKLIST

Take a good look at your staff and decide which people might work well together.

THE GAME PLAN

With everyone working together as a team, you'll have one working unit that will promote quality and production in your business. Many salons fail because the manager/owner uses an autocratic form of leadership, not allowing his team to make any decisions or participate in any operations in the salon. A busy manager or owner cannot do everything by him- or herself and must be able to delegate some of the work and authority. This gives the staff a feeling of belonging. Group delegation, or "team effort," is great because people who are pulling together to accomplish a goal don't want to let any of their team members down. General attendance seems to improve, and people tend to try harder in order not to be the "bad guy."

Begin by assigning small tasks to the team. Have a team decorate the salon, and put each person in charge of a special project in order to get the job done. Make the assignments simple and easy to understand. You act as a coach. This encourages coordination of the team members. Before long your staff will assume those responsibilities permanently, giving you a break and them a boost in their self-esteem.

Some of the benefits of group responsibility are:

1. Problem solving is put on a level where firsthand knowledge is more readily available.
2. The more tedious jobs can be distributed among several members of the staff.
3. Antagonism toward the bosses is minimized.
4. Supervisors who provide guidance for the team can devote extra time to more pressing matters.
5. Members are less willing to let the team down. Some people are less likely to be absent or late because they know others are depending upon them.

Teamwork is so important to your operation. With everyone acting as his or her own boss, many quarrels and misunderstandings are avoided. When teamwork is lacking in your salon, usually the productivity and quality of work suffer, and customers can feel it. You end up with a lot of turnover because the staff is not happy.

TIPS

- *Make sure you praise your people for their short-term successes.*
- *THERE IS A LOT OF WORK TO BE DONE. PICK YOUR TEAMS AND PLAY BALL!*

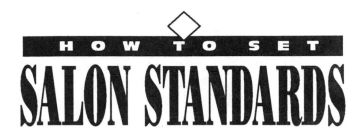

HOW TO SET
SALON STANDARDS

Most big corporations have standards that employees must follow. This is just as important for a salon. Without a standard against which to measure them, it is difficult to control and make decisions about your employees.

PREPARATION CHECKLIST

Set a goal to have the finest operation in town.

THE GAME PLAN

Some standards that should be set for every salon are:
1. The quality of work that you require.
2. Required technical training and examinations.
3. Required working hours and number of days off.
4. Standards for absenteeism.
5. Cost factors involved in products used.
6. The teamwork you've developed throughout your system.
7. The handling of special projects.
8. Pay structure — how employees will be paid, where they should be at a given point in time, and all the goals toward which they should strive in order to meet your standards.
9. Educational requirements.

If they know and understand all of these standards, at evaluation time you can measure their productivity against those standards. This makes it much easier to evaluate fairly whether or not they will be successful in your operation. If your staff has no model to compare themselves to, they won't be able to measure their progress, and you will have a chaotic organization. By setting standards, you can keep the quality of your skills as high as you want them.

TIPS

- *SET YOUR STANDARDS HIGH. IT WILL GIVE YOUR STAFF SOMETHING TO WORK FOR, AND YOUR CLIENTS WILL APPRECIATE THE QUALITY OF SERVICE!*

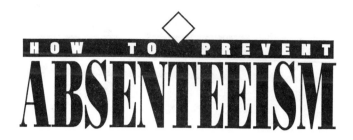

HOW TO PREVENT ABSENTEEISM

Absenteeism is a problem every salon has to deal with at one time or another. From the rescheduling and inconvenience of clients, the added workload for receptionist and other designers, to client disappointment, anger, and sometimes a decision to go elsewhere, absenteeism can cause a lot of problems!

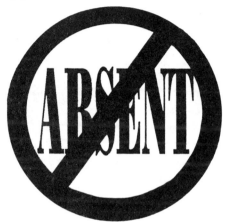

PREPARATION CHECKLIST

To tackle this problem, you need to think clearly, and you need to summon all of your authority and self-esteem. (This is sometimes necessary, but never fun.)

THE GAME PLAN

First, you must review existing policies and procedures. Analyze what works and what doesn't. Here are some restrictions to consider. These can be posted, and potential employees can be made aware of these rules at the time of hiring.

1. Any employee taking more than three days of sick leave in a row must bring a note from a doctor stating the cause of illness and indicating when he or she will be fit to return to work.
2. Any employee taking sick leave who does not call in before scheduled hours will be penalized one day's pay.
3. The management must be notified at least thirty days in advance of scheduled vacation time.
4. Vacation or sick days cannot accumulate beyond one year.

5. Anyone displaying chronic absenteeism will have his or her clients scheduled with other designers in the shop.

The following are some steps that can be taken at the time of disciplinary action:

1. Oral warning.
2. Written warning, with a copy placed in the employee's personnel file.
3. Postponement of any salary review for six months.
4. Docking of pay (one, two, or three days, depending upon previous disciplinary action).
5. Final step — dismissal for cause.

On the other hand, make it a point to reward an employee who has excellent attendance. Some suggestions are: additional paid time off, tickets to a show, or a dinner for two. Most important, don't forget to mention this in your salary review.

TIPS

- *Remember, when you find yourself in the uncomfortable position of having to deal with someone's absenteeism, it is not only your business that is at stake, but the morale of your clients and your other employees.*
- *If you have an employee who has reformed, reinforce the positive behavior. Don't let him or her slip back into old behavior patterns.*
- *MAY YOU HAVE THE ONE SALON THAT NEVER HAS THIS PROBLEM!*
- *RESPECT YOUR PEOPLE, AND THEY WILL RESPECT YOU!*

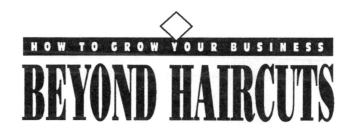

HOW TO GROW YOUR BUSINESS
BEYOND HAIRCUTS

This is an explosive time to be in the beauty business, because beauty goes so far beyond hairstyling. Today, both men and women are interested in being healthy and fit as well as physically attractive from head to toe.

PREPARATION CHECKLIST

Where do your interests lie? How about your finances, your education, and, most importantly, your determination? You can go as far in this industry today as your desires will take you!

THE GAME PLAN

A great hair design is only the beginning. Consider offering any or all of the following services:

1. Makeup — from the most conservative to the unusual.
2. Manicuring and pedicuring — traditional services that are more in demand today than ever!
3. Perm and color specialties — from your designers, who keep up with the latest trends from all over the world.
4. The finest in skin care — from relaxing facials to waxing and electrolysis.
5. Tanning — with guidance from your people to show your clients how to get the deepest tan while keeping their skin soft and supple.
6. Body toning — including aerobics for cardiovascular fitness and yoga for stretching and soothing.
7. Relaxation techniques — such as massage therapy, stress reduction, whirlpool, sauna, and steam baths.
8. Nutritional guidance — not only for weight reduction, but for general health and well-being. (Remember, some people are underweight.)
9. The latest methods for easing the body and mind, such as aroma therapy, reflexology, and acupressure.

These are just some of the possibilities available to you for expanding your business. Use your imagination — but remember, you cannot be successful without serious long-range planning, setting goals, and roadmapping!

TIPS

- *GATHER YOUR IDEAS, YOUR BEST PEOPLE, AND DEVISE A WAY. YOU ARE ONLY LIMITED BY YOUR MIND! BELIEVE IN WHAT YOU CAN DO AND IT'S YOURS! GO FOR IT!!*

HOW TO DETERMINE CRITICAL
STEPS FOR GROWTH

A salon has a life of its own, and life is never stagnant. If you are not moving forward (growth), then you are moving backward, and backward movement is a death sentence for your business.

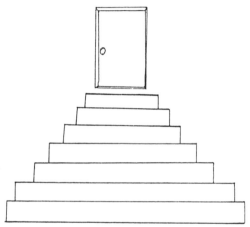

PREPARATION CHECKLIST

To prepare for this "exercise," you must be willing to take a long, honest look at yourself, for growth is a choice each individual must make for him- or herself.

THE GAME PLAN

It is crucially important that we are aware of our shortcomings so that we don't jump into a situation that we cannot handle. How do we find out what our shortcomings are? Here are some common possibilities:

1. Lack of knowledge.
2. Lack of skills.
3. Personality conflicts.
4. Situational misfit.
5. Limited ability.
6. Need more experience.

Once they are identified, you have choices to make. You can accept your shortcomings and do something about them, or you can deny them and face the consequences. Either way, you have made a choice over which you have control. You rarely have control, however, over consequences that result from your choices.

To build new strengths, you must find situations where learning is essential. Find ways to get help and support while you are learning. Anticipate a situation by asking questions, seeking advice or counseling, spending more time learning about the job, or using others' expertise and asking their opinions and help. You can also compensate for shortcomings by avoiding situations or delegating a job to others who can do it better. It is important to choose a staff who can compensate for your weaknesses. Another choice can be changing a situation totally by going into a new environment.

We can change ourselves by intensive counseling or coaching, personally changing ourselves, or changing just enough to get by.

Any way you look at it, change is the name of the game. Without change, there is no growth, and, as was stated in the beginning, without growth, there is death — to an individual and to a business.

TIPS

- *Remember that going through difficult changes builds character in a person. Such growth will make you stronger and better able to handle tough obstacles in the future.*
- *Some changes are more difficult to make than others, but circumstances are always neutral — and if you choose to go into a situation with a positive outlook, changes will seem to come more easily.*
- *MAKE GROWING AN ADVENTURE!*

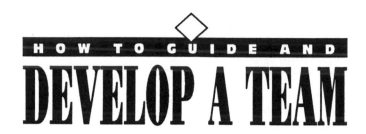

HOW TO GUIDE AND
DEVELOP A TEAM

You can hire fantastically talented designers, but if they can't work together, you can have more trouble than treasure. In this section, we are going to examine ways to make a lot of "loose parts" into a smoothly functioning unit.

PREPARATION CHECKLIST

In order to put "the game plan" into action, you must know your people.

THE GAME PLAN

Teaching your staff to work together and communicate is the basis for making them into a high-energy team. There are five building blocks, "the five T's," which you can use to accomplish this.

1. "Telling," or sharing decision-making. There are a variety of ways to get your message across about any subject. Most of these fall into one or more of five different leadership styles based on the situation and to whom you are talking. These leadership styles are:
   a. Autocratic — absolute supremacy, when you have absolute authority and hand out orders without question.
   b. Consultative — you retain the authority, but allow those under you some participation to express their opinions. You make the decisions, then ask for feedback.
   c. Participative — you share a common goal and work together to achieve it. You present a decision that is subject to change. This is especially good for situations that directly concern the staff.
   d. Democratic — ruled by the team members. Allow the staff the responsibility of handling the task from start to finish. You establish the limitations.
   e. Laissez-faire — hands off. You have complete trust in an individual or group to get the job done without your input.
2. Trust — empowerment of your staff. This gives your staff a feeling of importance. There are four keys to this "T."
   a. Feed their self-esteem.
   b. Listen and respond to their needs.
   c. Ask your staff for help.
   d. Offer help when you can, but do not assume the responsibility of the job.

16

3. Talking — the importance of communication. Don't close your mind to what your staff has to say.
4. Teaching and training — development of yourself and others.
5. Taking care — treating others the way you want to be treated. With a plan like this, you can build a team that is dynamic and non-stoppable!

TIPS

- *It is so important that you LISTEN to your staff. If they were worthy of hiring, they are worthy of hearing.*
- *RESPECT YOUR PEOPLE AND THEY WILL RESPECT YOU!*

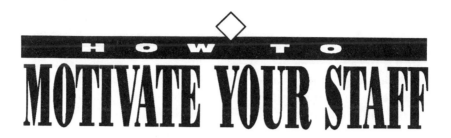

MOTIVATE YOUR STAFF

Did you ever say, "I wish I could motivate my staff," meaning, "I wish I could get them to do a better job."? This is not difficult, but the real motivation starts with you.

PREPARATION CHECKLIST

In order to accomplish this, you must have a clear idea of what you want from your staff and be able to communicate it to them in a way that they cannot misunderstand.

THE GAME PLAN

First of all, you should be a model for your employees. Approach your work with a sense of urgency and pride. Use your time efficiently, and meet your deadlines. Most importantly, set goals for yourself and your salon, and try very hard to accomplish them. Show your employees by your actions that the job you do really matters and that quality and service are the keys to success in our industry.

Ask for performance. Give your employees job descriptions detailing their responsibilities. Find out what they can contribute to the company in addition to the tasks on their job descriptions. Do they have artistic or writing abilities, decorating skills? Ask them to make a commitment to contribute some of this extra talent as you need it, or allow them to be creative.

Give lots of positive reinforcement to your staff, and don't take acceptable work for granted. Thank them, and commend them on a job well done. Every time they make an improvement, let them know that you notice. Draw smiley faces on their goal sheets or paychecks when they do well. Compliment them at a staff meeting or on the floor. When a team member does an exceptional job, applaud him publicly.

Build relationships with your employees. Take an interest in their wants and needs. Treat them as you would want to be treated, with kindness, respect, and trust that their intentions are good. Do things with them as a group, such as picnics, bowling, skiing, etc. Try to build them as a team instead of just individuals. Ask for their opinions, and listen to their points of view. Keep an open mind, and you will find that people are more likely to cooperate when changes need to be made.

Refuse to accept poor performance. Everyone needs to be reprimanded or coached sometime in his career. Try to be encouraging when you correct someone. This demonstrates to your people that standards matter. It is better to aim for perfection and hit excellence than to aim for good and hit average.

18

TIPS

- *Don't expect people to respect you just because you're there. Work to earn their respect, and be the example.*
- *Personalize your praise. Don't say, "Your dress is pretty." Say, "You look pretty in that dress."*
- *BE POSITIVE, AND YOU WILL HAVE A POSITIVE STAFF!*

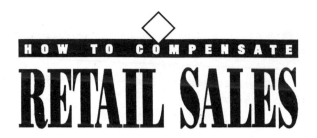

RETAIL SALES

After you have successfully trained your staff to sell your products, the most important motivator is the "incentive."

PREPARATION CHECKLIST

What will be their reward for selling? It's time to make a decision.

THE GAME PLAN

Here are some suggestions.

1. A percentage of the sale. The standard rate for this is between 10 and 15 percent, and it can be paid monthly, quarterly, yearly, or any way that works well for your business.
2. Contests are a great way to get your staff excited about selling. Give away a prize for the highest sales or percentage of sales.

TIPS

- *Remember, when choosing an incentive gift, "One person's pleasure is another's poison." If the prize you're giving does not interest some members of your staff, chances are they will not work very hard to attain their selling goals.*
- *Incentive programs should be creative and fun, but the main benefit to your staff will be in their paychecks and self-esteem, for they are not only selling products, they are selling themselves, their skills, and their services.*
- *SHOW YOUR STAFF THE VALUE OF SALES, AND WATCH THEM GO!*

HOW TO DO
NON MONETARY REWARDS

In the work situation, most people respond positively when the boss recognizes them and gives them praise. They will work harder if they know they are appreciated and if they are learning new skills.

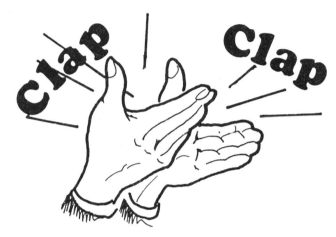

PREPARATION CHECKLIST

Every week, try to find someone in your salon who could use a little recognition.

THE GAME PLAN

Find a way to acknowledge a job well done. Shake an employee's hand or pat him or her on the back and say that you appreciate a great job last week or that he or she met the weekly goals and you are very proud. Another idea, if your salon or corporation is large, is to have an awards banquet. Present awards for such things as good attendance, good attitude, or most promising employee in your company. A diploma or small trophy isn't costly and means a lot. You can also buy small tokens of appreciation for length of service a staff member has given to the company, such as a watch, a desk clock, or a pen and pencil set. If you have a company newsletter, choose an employee of the week or month to write about, or hang that person's picture up. Treat a staff member to breakfast or lunch, take people out on their birthdays, or award someone with a dinner for two. Give someone a call. Let him or her know that you care and you appreciate what he or she has done for you. Or just say thank you. That's all that most people want to hear, and it can encourage extra effort in the future.

TIPS

- *RECOGNITION OR APPLAUSE COSTS NOTHING, SO GIVE IT OUT FREELY. YOUR PEOPLE WILL THINK YOU ARE THE BEST BOSS, AND THEIR PERFORMANCE WILL SHOW IT!*

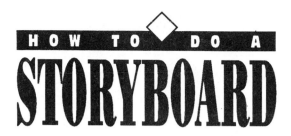

STORYBOARD

Storyboarding is a term used by advertising agencies and artists who draw pictures that form stories. Cartoons are a form of storyboarding. Television ads are put together this way. Walt Disney started Disneyland by forming pictures on paper that led to his dream, his vision, his reality.

Storyboarding can be an incredible way to create an idea or a promotion, develop customer services, or form goals for yourself and your salon. Writing things down and seeing pictures can help crystallize your thoughts and lead you down the path to success!

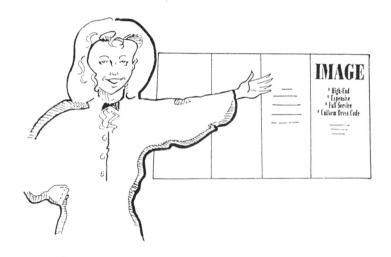

PREPARATION CHECKLIST

1. Chalk or whiteboard, flip chart, or long sheets of paper.
2. Chalk or magic markers.

THE GAME PLAN

First, list the subjects you would like to discuss; for instance: image, goals, educational sessions, staff participation. Each person involved can contribute a word or a few words directly related to that subject. Don't allow any discussion or negative ideas at this time. Encourage everyone to participate. Here are two examples:

IMAGE	EDUCATION
Upscale	Haircutting class with someone well-known
Professional	Retail class
High technical skills	Outside guest artist
Creative	Basic perm class
Uniform dressing	Classes regularly

After you have covered all of your topics, put them together and form a picture of what you should be doing to direct yourself toward the goals described on the storyboard. List the costs, the goals, their importance, and a time frame in which to achieve them. Delegate jobs to people who can carry them out, then just see that they get done!

TIPS

- *This procedure can be used in many situations in your everyday life as well as your business. Don't forget to consider it whenever you're planning for anything.*
- *STORYBOARDING CAN BE THE BEGINNING OF NEW AND EXCITING ADDITIONS TO YOUR SALON BUSINESS!*

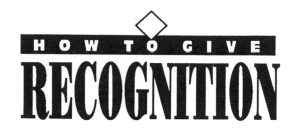

HOW TO GIVE
RECOGNITION

As owners or managers, we sometimes get so involved in supervising, planning, and financing our salons that we forget to acknowledge those who really make it all happen — our staff!

PREPARATION CHECKLIST

During your salon evaluations, ask your staff to express their feelings about your management style and about what they feel they need or want from you. I think you'll find that most people want recognition for their accomplishments, support in their work, and a general feeling that they matter to you and your business.

THE GAME PLAN

Make a point each day to find something good to say to each one of your staff. Most people respond to praise so much more positively than they do to fault-finding. Reward them for their efforts. Here are some things you might do:

1. Remember birthdays with a rosebud, a card, or even just a telephone call if you have more than one salon.
2. Include your staff in the decision-making processes at your monthly staff meetings. Take them out occasionally for breakfast or dinner meetings. It will make them feel special.
3. Have a staff photo session. Let everyone bring models to be photographed, and display the shots in your salon.
4. Delegate jobs to your people beyond their jobs as hairdressers. Involve them in projects that will help you, and at the same time make them feel that they are an important part of the shop's success. Examples:
   a. Decoration committee: These people will be responsible for decorating the salon for holidays and special occasions. They can also design your retail and boutique item displays.
   b. Newsletter: If one of your staff has some writing ability, let him or her be the news reporter for your salon newsletter.
   c. Education director: Appoint someone who is a good teacher to set up an educational program for your staff.

      d. Promotions committee: These staff members can create and encourage staff participation in outside promotional ideas such as shows, cut-a-thons, or make-overs.

5. Allow your staff to put on a show at a nightclub or do a charity benefit. This allows them to be creative. Give them guidelines and a budget, and watch them roll!

TIPS

- *Make it a habit to make a positive comment to every member of your staff each day. Let them know that they are important to you.*
- *REMEMBER, AN APPRECIATED EMPLOYEE IS A HARD-WORKING AND LOYAL EMPLOYEE!*

HOW TO PREPARE FOR
YOUR EVALUATIONS

In order for your working relationship with your staff to be most successful, it's important to evaluate each employee's performance at least once a year. This can also be a time to allow employees to evaluate your leadership qualities. Both parties will learn and grow if this is handled in an impartial and professional manner.

PREPARATION CHECKLIST

1. Computer sheet with the following information:
   a. List of service and retail goals.
   b. Service dollars — average service dollars per client.
   c. Retail dollars — average retail dollars per client.
   d. Percentage of goals met.
   e. Timesheet — hours worked and time off.
   f. Breakdown of services completed.
   g. Client retention sheet/lost client report.
   h. Cost analysis on each designer.
2. Information sheets with the following information:
   a. Extra job assignments.
   b. Improvements or suggestions given.
   c. Outside public relations for designer.
   d. Training classes.

THE GAME PLAN

Hold your meetings in a quiet, private place where you will be uninterrupted, and set aside at least an hour for each employee. Have your evaluation forms completed in advance. Ask your people to fill out evaluation forms on management and bring them along.

Be prepared with a list of topics you want to cover. Discuss problems in each category and how they might be solved and, more importantly, PRAISE your people for a job well done. Encourage them to growth and success. And don't forget to ask them how you can improve your management skills.

TIPS

- *Make sure the purpose of the interview is clearly understood. Most employees are not aware of how their work is evaluated or what appraisals are all about. Let them know what they are being evaluated on, and then stick to the essential points in the review session.*

- *Keep the purpose simple — to help each employee work closer to potential. Anything that may help an employee achieve this should be brought out in the review.*

- *Conduct the review as an exchange of information, not as a report card. Remember, the evaluation form is only a tool. List all the individual's strengths and weaknesses and discuss them. There is little chance for advancement unless both parties can agree when improvement is needed and how to deal with it. Conducting your interview as an exchange of information is an indication that you are willing to work together.*

- *Stick to essentials. One way to stay focused is to let your employee know ahead of time the topics of discussion. Some good examples are: job proficiency, working relationships with other team members, and accomplishment of goals set at the last evaluation. Also, have the employee inform you in advance of his or her concerns, so you can be prepared. The seven questions that most employees want answered are:*
  1. *How am I doing?*
  2. *How can I improve?*
  3. *Is there an opportunity for advancement?*
  4. *What will be expected of me before the next review?*
  5. *How will my work be evaluated during that time?*
  6. *What kind of assistance or attention can I expect from the supervisor?*
  7. *What changes are likely in our operation in the months ahead, and how will they affect me?*

- *Organize your approach. A lot of supervisors find the "RAP" review useful:*
  REVIEW the past.
  ANALYZE the present.
  PLAN the future.
  If the goal is truly to help an individual work up to potential, discussion of the past and present is mainly beneficial in helping plan for the future. Proportionately, spend about 25 percent of the time on the past, 15 percent on the present, and 60 percent on the future.

TRAPS

- *Don't dwell on negatives. Take a positive approach to problem solving, and people will respond positively.*

- *Don't get defensive if your employee offers constructive criticism of your management skills. Remember that everyone can stand to improve something, and maybe one of his suggestions will make your life easier! Working together is an indication of your willingness to be a helper and not just a drill sergeant.*

- *BE WILLING TO LISTEN, AND EMPLOYEES WILL BE WILLING TO LEARN!*

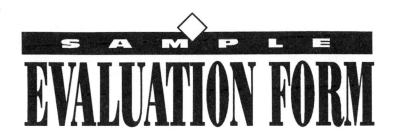

EVALUATION FORM

I. GOALS
    A. Quarterly target goal — services. .... _____
    B. Service goal obtained for period. .... _____
    C. Percentage of service quota for designated period. .... _____
    D. Average service dollars per client. .... _____
    E. Quarterly target goal — retail. .... _____
    F. Retail goal obtained for period. .... _____
    G. Percentage of retail quota for designated period. .... _____
    H. Average retail dollars per client. .... _____

II. CLIENTS SERVICED AND LOST
    A. Total number of clients serviced. .... _____
    B. Total number of clients repeated. .... _____
    C. Total number of new clients. .... _____
    D. Total number of lost clients. .... _____
    E. Percentage lost clients to new. .... _____
    F. Personal goals achieved. .... _____

III. HOURS
    A. Number of hours scheduled to work for period. .... _____
    B. Number of actual hours worked. .... _____
    C. Number of days off — vacation, sick, etc. .... _____
    D. Total monies per hour to salon. .... _____
    E. Total hours divided into total service = ... _____

IV. TECHNICAL SKILLS
    A. Haircutting skills 1 2 3 4 5 6
    B. Color skills 1 2 3 4 5 6
    C. Perm skills 1 2 3 4 5 6
    D. Relaxer skills 1 2 3 4 5 6
    E. Manicuring skills 1 2 3 4 5 6
    F. Overall quality of work 1 2 3 4 5 6
    G. Salesmanship 1 2 3 4 5 6
    H. Initiative to learn 1 2 3 4 5 6

MANAGEMENT

    I. Initiative to make goals 1 2 3 4 5 6

    J. Working to capacity 1 2 3 4 5 6

V. TIMING

    A. Average time for haircut and style 1 2 3 4 5 6

    B. Average time for perm 1 2 3 4 5 6

    C. Average time for color 1 2 3 4 5 6

    D. Average time for highlights 1 2 3 4 5 6

VI. ATTITUDE

    A. Appropriate behavior 1 2 3 4 5 6

    B. Appearance 1 2 3 4 5 6

    C. Professional attitude toward clients and teammates 1 2 3 4 5 6

    D. Attendance 1 2 3 4 5 6

    E. Punctuality 1 2 3 4 5 6

    F. Teamwork 1 2 3 4 5 6

    G. Attitude towards management 1 2 3 4 5 6

    H. Constructive criticism 1 2 3 4 5 6

VII. SALON MAINTENANCE

    A. Neatness of station 1 2 3 4 5 6

    B. Floor supervisor's job 1 2 3 4 5 6

    C. General salon duties 1 2 3 4 5 6

VIII. ADDITIONAL RESPONSIBILITIES

    Assignments inside or outside the salon; examples:

    decorating, writing, teaching a class, etc. 1 2 3 4 5 6

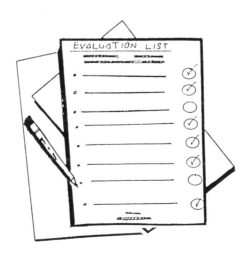

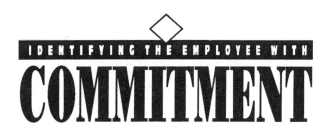

IDENTIFYING THE EMPLOYEE WITH
COMMITMENT

Some employees will work hard from the minute they start. They show up for work no matter what their health. They're seldom late or absent, and they continue to work under the most difficult circumstances. Sometimes these people have to be told to go home when they're sick. These are committed, dedicated employees.

PREPARATION CHECKLIST

You don't need to prepare for this one. You just need to be extremely lucky or be such a perfect boss that potential employees will be knocking down your door to come and dedicate their careers to you!

THE GAME PLAN

You never know how or when you are going to get a hard-working, committed person. Applicant testing to find someone with these qualities has not been successful. Some personnel experts believe that personality traits indicating a higher than average drive for success could be an indicator. You can also try contacting a previous supervisor to discuss an applicant's work habits, but only with permission from the applicant. The attributes to look for in the hard-working person are:

1. Quality — the worker strives very hard for accuracy, has good technical ability, and is a perfectionist. He or she has a very low tolerance for making mistakes.
2. Punctuality — the person is usually early and never keeps clients waiting, continuously striving for timeliness and perfection.
3. Responsibility — he or she rarely makes excuses for not completing an assignment and takes few personal breaks. This is the person who has to be sent home when he or she is sick.
4. Diligence and a drive for success — he or she is always ready to work overtime without complaint, working as late or as long as you wish, and never turning down a client.
5. Productivity — the applicant has very high standards and strives to surpass any goals set by management.
6. An insatiable desire to learn — he or she wants to know everything there is to know. This person reads and studies everything that can lead to growth on the job.

Some of the good work habits of the committed worker can be imitated by others, especially younger employees. Assign some of these people to watch or work with this person as a mentor. This can positively affect their work behavior and increase their productivity.

TIPS

- *To keep the committed worker happy, increase his or her responsibilities. Assign something difficult to accomplish, with a deadline. Be reasonable, of course.*
- *DON'T FORGET TO APPRECIATE AND COMPLIMENT YOUR MOST VALUABLE EMPLOYEES!*

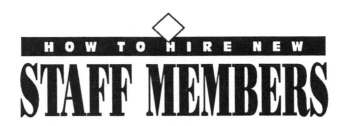

HOW TO HIRE NEW
STAFF MEMBERS

Selecting staff members for your team is one of the most important things you'll do for your business. It is well worth the effort to spend enough time in the interviewing process to make sure you hire the kind of people you can trust to do the job.

PREPARATION CHECKLIST

Once again, in preparation for this task you need a clear mind.

THE GAME PLAN

Begin with a plan outlining the kind of person you want to work for you. Draft a job description including all job criteria — quality of work, technical skills required, salesmanship abilities, training and education expected, number of years experience preferred, work hours, and salary. Also consider things like personality, initiative, attitude, goals, desire for additional training and/or promotions, and team spirit.

You need to know what kind of salon you want. If you are planning a very expensive and elite salon, you must make sure that the people you hire are able to meet the demands of that clientele. If a children's shop is what you have in mind, your employees should be very patient and love kids.

A vital point to remember is that your staff should be a team. Choosing people who you think can work well together is a major consideration.

TIPS

- *Don't necessarily hire someone just because he or she has a large clientele. If he doesn't get along with the others, you have lost more than you could gain.*
- *Try to schedule your interviews for after closing time. You will have fewer interruptions, less chance of embarrassment with existing staff members, and, if your prospective employee has a job elsewhere, he or she will be finished for the day. It will be convenient for both of you, and you will be more able to concentrate on the interview.*
- *TRUST YOUR INSTINCTS TO HELP YOU HIRE THE BEST!*

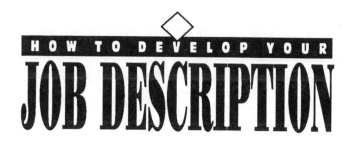

HOW TO DEVELOP YOUR
JOB DESCRIPTION

A job description is essential in order to make clear the responsibilities of the position to the applicant.

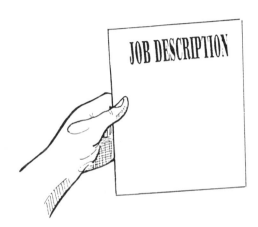

JOB DESCRIPTION

PREPARATION CHECKLIST

Know what you expect of your designers and what you will do for them.

THE GAME PLAN

Here is a sample job description. You can adapt it to fit the requirements of your business.

POSITION: Designer   **GRADE LEVEL:** 1

SALON: Your Business Name

REPORTING TO: Salon Manager or Training Staff Member

PRIMARY DUTIES OF POSITION: You must:

1. Consult with client(s); offer advice and suggestions regarding their hair-care needs. Know current styles and fashion. Continue education regarding current trends in styling, and be able to perform these current styles on clients.
2. Know perm techniques used in the salon. Know the types of perms used in salon.
3. Know the basics of hair color and the product knowledge regarding the colors used in the salon. Know how to highlight hair with foils, using salon techniques.
4. Have training and ability to perform cuts and styling techniques on all kinds, textures, and lengths of hair.

5. Know names, uses, and correct applications of all retail products carried in salon.
6. Provide excellent customer service through consultations, consistent quality of work, time schedules, awareness of comforts, educating clients on how to take care of their hair, and suggesting retail products for them to use at home.
7. Have necessary tools to do job. (See manager.)
8. Meet or exceed revenue quotas; participate in any salon promotions geared to attract new clients; actively seek prospective clients through outside sources, promos, friends, or family referrals.

ADDITIONAL DUTIES: You must:
1. Perform any assigned cleaning duties within the salon as a team member or floor supervisor.
2. Be willing to accept responsibility for salon projects, such as teaching a class, doing a fashion show, doing a marketing assignment within or outside the scope of normal working hours.
3. Help teammates when they are in need, and accept responsibilities for duties that may be assigned by management when necessary.

REQUIREMENTS: Current cosmetology license

PRIMARY SALON RESPONSIBILITIES

Professional attitude

Professional appearance

Career oriented

Service oriented

Technically proficient

Sales ability

Product knowledge

Personal and salon hygiene

Listening ability

Consultation

Creativity

Hair-cutting skills

Perming knowledge

Coloring knowledge

Need awareness

ADDITIONAL SALON RESPONSIBILITIES

Inventory

Marketing

Public speaking and consulting

Media and public relations

Quality control

Office — data processing

Direct mail

Recruiting

Cleaning

Errands

Front desk

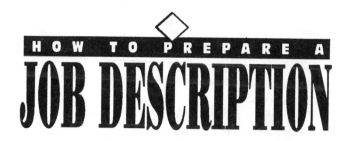

HOW TO PREPARE A
JOB DESCRIPTION

A job description is a statement that clarifies the requirements of the position for which you are hiring. It defines the employee's responsibilities and is a communication tool between employee and employer. It should be written so that it will prevent misunderstandings about what is expected from the employee and what will be provided by the employer. It should include the qualifications required for the job, the responsibilities, major working relationships, and opportunities for promotion.

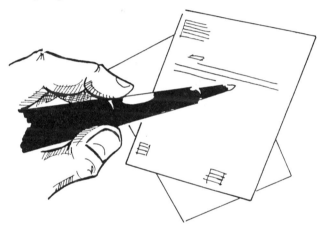

PREPARATION CHECKLIST

Before you begin, you must think about what is expected of the applicant and what you are willing to give.

THE GAME PLAN

Here is a sample format. It contains some ideas to consider when you draw up your own job descriptions.

1. Job title.
2. Level or rank.
3. Job definition — summary of type of job.
4. Location.
5. Manager's name.
6. Starting salary range.
   a. Overtime salary.

    b. Bonus incentive plans.

7. Hours — number & times.

8. Working conditions.

Qualifications

1. License from school, college, degrees, classes, advanced courses taken or any other type of training.

2. Experience — general and specific work experience and/or management experience.

3. Specialized skills required — typing, computer skills, hair coloring, perms, etc.

Responsibilities

1. Duties — describe all job functions and areas of responsibility. Allow space for adding new projects, changes, or extra assignments.

2. Tools and/or equipment required before starting the job.

3. Training required to maintain position.

4. Goals.

Working Relationships

1. Employee's supervisor.

2. Those whom the employee supervises.

3. Contacts.

Promotions

1. Possibilities within present position.

2. Positions available in the future.

3. Outside promotions booked by salon.

4. Promotion policy concerning pay increases.

TIPS

- *Make sure you spell everything out clearly. Sometimes what you think is obvious or not worth mentioning can be a cause for confusion to someone else.*

- *HIGHLIGHT THE POSITIVE ASPECTS, AND GOOD PEOPLE WILL LINE UP AT THE DOOR!*

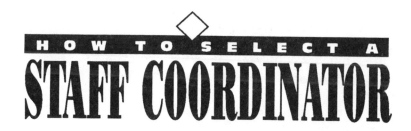

HOW TO SELECT A
STAFF COORDINATOR

A staff coordinator is the person who represents the staff members as a spokesperson to management. He can be a great asset to the salon owner, especially if you have a large staff of people. Instead of having a lot of people coming to you at any time with their problems and concerns, you have one representative and a lot more order.

PREPARATION CHECKLIST

Take inventory of your staff. You want to choose a person who listens well, has organizational skills, gets along well with others, and has the ability to develop creative solutions to problems.

THE GAME PLAN

When selecting a staff coordinator, you need to consider who you feel can handle the many responsibilities. They will include attending your regular staff/management meetings, where the coordinator will address the needs of the staff, offer salon improvement suggestions, and bring ideas and solutions. The coordinator will hold staff meetings without management present to discuss staff interests. The subjects usually covered are inside and outside educational opportunities, goals, new services, how to handle assistants and how they are performing, customer services, super services that staff would like to offer to their clients, and new ideas and suggestions that they might like to incorporate into the salon. The coordinator can collect educational materials and make sure the staff is aware of upcoming shows and classes.

A staff coordinator is a great way to get feedback from your people and become aware of their desires and concerns.

TIPS

- *Your staff coordinator is someone who could easily become your "right arm." Choose someone who you and your employees can trust.*
- *Allow your staff a lot of input when making this decision. After all, this person will be their representative.*
- *A FAIR-MINDED STAFF COORDINATOR WILL KEEP ORDER AND GOOD WILL IN YOUR BUSINESS RELATIONSHIPS!*
- *HAPPY HUNTING!*

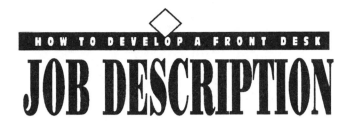

JOB DESCRIPTION

A job description is essential for this position, which really involves customer relations. It will help you determine what qualities to look for when hiring, and it will give the employee a complete description of what is expected of the person in this position.

PREPARATION CHECKLIST

Know what you expect from your customer relations person, and what he or she can expect from you.

THE GAME PLAN

Here are some ideas about what to include in a job description for your customer relations person. You will probably add and subtract things as they pertain to your business.

1. Open the salon at least fifteen minutes before the first client arrives. Can include: lights, computer start-up, coffee preparation, getting clients' robes ready, turning on music, opening files, readying cash drawer, giving designers the client slips, and turning on heat or air.
2. Proper dress code.
3. Phone procedures — how to book appointments and handle complaints; personal calls for designers and other employees (when to interrupt a client's service with a personal call); how to sell extra services on the phone ("Would you like a manicure with your haircut?"); call backs and reminders to clients; and telemarketing procedures.
4. Retail arrangements — This may include commissions, credit, how and when to stock shelves, shipment arrivals, c.o.d. deliveries, prices, computerized inventory control, discounts and special promotions, orders, etc.
5. Booking procedures — times and names of designers and other staff; how much time each designer needs for each service; who does what; price structure; fair booking practices; list of things that some staff members can't do (if necessary); and how to fill in appointment book.
6. Customer relations — what to do with a brand new client; what to say and do when a designer is running late; low-key selling; client conversation; rebooking clients, etc.
7. Free services — family, friends, each other; how to handle tips.

8. Money transactions — computer check-out; receipts; refund policy; charge cards; check policies; making change; cash float requirements; banking procedures; bill paying; check writing; cash advances; payroll; etc.

9. End of workday — balancing drawer; procedures for computerized or manual salon; what should be done with the money; preparation for next day; lockup; etc.

10. Benefits — vacations; insurances (health and workman's compensation); paid holidays; special requests; etc.

11. Time and conduct requirements — attendance; lunch policy; hours; absenteeism; staff meetings; outside educationals; proper conduct; making clients feel at home; pleasant telephone voice; and, above all — SMILE!

TIPS

- *Have small envelopes with "To:" and "From:" printed on them in which clients can leave tips at the desk.*
- *Be very thorough and precise when describing job requirements. Don't assume anything. Don't leave room for, "I didn't know that was part of my job."*
- *APPRECIATE THE VALUE OF THIS EMPLOYEE!*

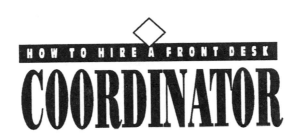

HOW TO HIRE A FRONT DESK
COORDINATOR

The person who handles your front desk will leave an indelible mark on each of your clients — not only of herself, but of you and your salon as well. Make sure he or she is making an impression that is an asset to your business.

PREPARATION CHECKLIST

Know the type of person for whom you are looking. Make up a job description and find a person who fits it.

THE GAME PLAN

Once you have written a job description, you can begin looking for the right person. Advertise in the newspaper or local magazines. Don't begin with "Receptionist wanted," but ask for "Customer relations person" or "Customer service person." These people have had experience with customers' needs and wants. They know how to handle complaints and what to do when things are not right.

When you have identified a prospect, set up an interview. Reserve a special time and place when you will not be interrupted by calls or clients. Be as professional as you expect your potential employee to be. Have the individual fill out an application form, and take the time to look it over. And always check references. You should interview more than one person to give yourself a better perspective.

When you have decided to offer the job to someone, have him or her come back for a second interview. This interview should be more comprehensive and should provide the candidate with more specific information about the position, its responsibilities and benefits. This is also a good time to give a tour of the workplace, introduce your staff, and possibly set up an opportunity for staff and the candidate to ask each other questions. Finally, answer the candidate's questions about the job and/or the company. Then write an evaluation for future reference.

Here are some questions you might ask in an interview:

1. Tell me about your most recent job. What would you like to change? What did you like most and least about the job?
2. How do you feel you contributed to the organization in that position?
3. Why do you want to work in this field and for this company?
4. Do you prefer to work in groups or independently?
5. What has had a major impact on your development and abilities?

6. What situations did you find challenging?
7. How do you deal with pressure?
8. List your major strengths/unique characteristics.
9. Where do you want to be in five years? In ten years?

TIPS

- *If you do not have an office, consider having your interview in a restaurant or some other quiet place.*
- *HAPPY HUNTING!*

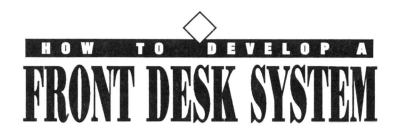

HOW TO DEVELOP A
FRONT DESK SYSTEM

Front desk operation can make or break your business. It must be run smoothly and efficiently, and to do so you need to determine exactly what you need in that area.

PREPARATION CHECKLIST

Take a long, serious look at your present system and decide how it could be improved to benefit salon procedures.

THE GAME PLAN

Ask yourself the following questions about your front desk system: What kind of telephone system is required, and where should you place extensions? Do you need an intercom? Do you have a pay phone located in a quiet place, so regular phone lines won't be tied up?

Is your desk large enough and capable of handling the number of people who work there? Does its location allow it to accommodate the traffic flow easily? Do you need more file space? Is your appointment book system right for your salon? Can everyone understand each other's codes?

Are you computerized or thinking about it? If so, do you have enough room for a terminal and printer? Can your staff handle computer procedures? Do you know how to read computer reports and use them to your benefit?

If you sell retail, is the retail rack close enough to the reception desk so your employees don't waste time running back and forth? Do you have bags for your products? If you sell boutique items, are they close enough to be shown easily? Are your displays cleaned and stocked daily? Are prices coded and marked clearly?

Do you have magazines available for clients? Are they related to fashion and hairstyles? Do you have men's fashion magazines and perhaps a *Newsweek* or a business magazine? Is your magazine rack neat and clean?

Do you have a place for clients to hang their coats and place their umbrellas? Do you have an adequate changing room?

Do you allow smoking in your salon? If so, be sure to have clean ashtrays available and, if not, make sure signs are clearly posted in the reception area and other places.

Do you have a stereo and/or VCR? Do the music and videos you play complement the clientele you serve? Are your speakers and screen placed for proper viewing and regulated sound, and are your controls at or near the front desk so the customer relations person can monitor everything? Do your videos relate to the fashion statement your salon is making, and are they changed periodically?

The answers to these questions can help you develop a system to fit your needs and prosper in your business.

TIPS

- *Unless you are independently wealthy, be sure to prioritize your needs and shop wisely.*
- *LET YOUR RECEPTION AREA MAKE A GREAT IMPRESSION!*

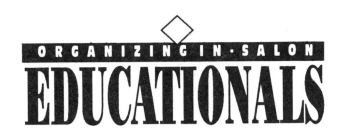

ORGANIZING IN-SALON EDUCATIONALS

Keeping your staff well-educated and up-to-date is very important. If they are not aware of current trends, they will surely get lost in the crowd.

PREPARATION CHECKLIST

Set aside at least one day a month for educationals. Schedule a day when the workload is light, and allow at least three hours for each session. Be creative when planning these classes. Perhaps one of your staff members has a skill to share with the others (see TIPS), or you might invite a member of a hair design team or an outside educator to speak. And don't limit yourself to techniques. Try motivational speakers, personality testing, and people who can teach your employees about teamwork and promoting themselves, their work, their workplace, and the products they sell. Role play with sales and service methods. Teach retailing. Use your imagination! Help your staff become successful, well-rounded, interesting people.

THE GAME PLAN

1. Set a specific day and time for your educationals.
2. Make sure your program is planned and prepared in advance. Have a lesson plan and all materials you will need ready to go. This includes any video equipment, visual aids, and work/information sheets you might want to distribute.
3. Inform your staff by posting a notice. If applicable, include a list of the things they will need to bring to the class (tools, implements, notebooks, etc.).
4. Designate a place in your salon for your classes, and have it ready with chairs set up for appropriate viewing and participation.
5. Allow time for questions and answers either during or after your presentation.
6. Follow your lesson plan to the best of your ability, and begin and end your class on time.

TIPS

- *Plan all educational sessions at least four to five months ahead of time.*
- *Don't be afraid to use an employee who is particularly talented in a specific area like color or perms, or even shampooing and massage, to share with the others. This will not only give valuable insight to the staff, but it will also give the "teacher" experience talking in front of people, which will, in turn, make it easier to talk to clients.*

- *Have staff members who have been to a show or have some knowledge of a new product, technique, or piece of equipment share with the others what they have learned.*
- *Call local colleges, hospitals, and businesses to find men and women who will speak to your staff about psychology, understanding people, sales skills, stress factors and how to deal with them, people skills, etc. You may be surprised at how rich in talented resources your town or city is.*
- *Ask your staff for their suggestions about what they would like to learn.*
- *Encourage all employees to attend each session. Make it a job requirement.*
- *If you have a large staff, consider gearing some classes to new people and others to experienced people.*
- *Stick to the schedule of classes you have planned.*
- *Keep the sessions interesting and simple. Don't bore people with old knowledge or confuse them with complicated presentations. You don't want to lose them!*
- *If possible, videotape all classes and keep them for future references. Anyone who missed a class or who wishes to see it again will be able to get the information. Remember, most people retain only 10 percent of what they hear! A videotape is a great way to give feedback to the speaker, which can help him or her improve teaching and/or selling skills.*
- *EDUCATION IS THE KEY! GO FOR IT!*

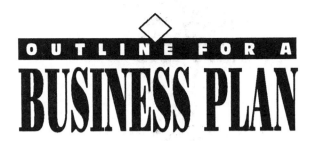

OUTLINE FOR A
BUSINESS PLAN

A business plan is like a road map. It helps you understand where you are, where you want to go, and how you are going to get there. It begins with a definition of the business and continues through the fundamental aspects of operations, projections, and plans.

Writing it down forces you to consider all the areas of importance in running your business. It can reveal the risks as well as the rewards. Used as a guide in decision making, it should describe all the functional aspects of the business in addition to the key financial areas. A business outline should also provide you with a document to show potential investors and financing institutions.

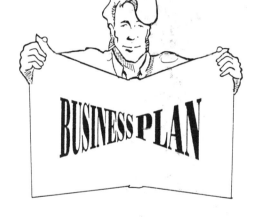

PREPARATION CHECKLIST

- *For this project, you will need information. Gather anything and everything you can find that deals with your business.*

THE GAME PLAN

The following is a suggested outline for a business plan. It is not written in stone. Use it as a guide, and adapt it to your needs.

  I. THE BUSINESS
     A. Description of the kind of salon you want to open
     B. Marketing strategy

    C. Management policies
    D. Personal plans
    E. Necessary insurance policies
    F. Financial plans
    G. Areas of growth

II. **FINANCIAL DATA**
    A. Loan application
    B. Investor's prospectus
    C. Financial statements — personal or other business
       1. Balance sheet
       2. Income statement
       3. Three-year projection
          a. First year — detail month by month
          b. Second & third years — by quarters
       4. Sources and uses of funds
       5. Cash flow statement
       6. Yearly budget
    D. Capital equipment list
    E. Breakeven analysis
    F. Financial reports for existing business
       1. Balance sheet for past three years
       2. Income statement for past three years
       3. Tax returns

III. **SUPPORTING DOCUMENTS**
    A. Personal biographies or resumes
    B. Owner's personal financial requirements and statements
    C. Cost-of-living budgets
    D. Credit reports
    E. Letters of reference
    F. Recommendations
    G. Copies of leases
    H. Contracts and legal documents

Developing the plan can be tricky if you've never done it before. Try getting a book on how to write a business plan at your library, or call the Small Business Association in your area for information.

TIPS

- *Seek the help of your lawyer, accountant, CPA, bookkeeper, and any friends who may provide you with the information that you need.*
- *USE EVERY RESOURCE AVAILABLE, AND GOOD LUCK!!*

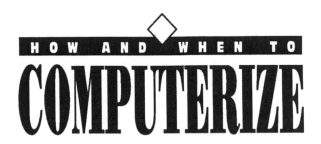

HOW AND WHEN TO
COMPUTERIZE

Computers are not just a passing fancy. They're accepted by most people as a common managerial tool, and today a business without computerization is at a distinct disadvantage. Computers are here to stay!

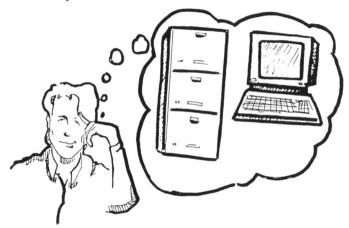

PREPARATION CHECKLIST

With careful consideration, take a long look at the way your business is currently running. Can you survive without computerizing? Please read on.

THE GAME PLAN

A computer will consolidate much of the business of running a salon. The first important attribute is that you can retrieve any information you put into it because of its built-in memory. Unlike human memory, it is almost unfailing, and, once it's told something, it doesn't forget. It can also move data around, making it possible to retrieve only the information you need. For instance, you can bring up a list of inventory supplies, every individual's performance breakdown, the day's receipts, or your profit and loss statements. You can list all of your clients and divide them into categories, such as those who haven't returned for a certain amount of time or those who work in a specific area.

Of course, your computer can only give you the information you put into it. Usually, this work is done by the person who manages your front desk.

Another advantage of a computer is its ability to calculate. It can run millions of computations in a second without error, and the playback can be on cards, sheets, or video screens.

To get the computer to do what you want it to do, it must be "programmed." The machine is given detailed instructions, called a "program," which is stored just like the data. If changes need to be made, the instructions are changed by the "programmer."

It is simpler and generally more effective to purchase a program suited to your operation than to try to create one yourself, and you should understand that not every chore can be automated. Automation is the answer to many problems, but you'll find in some cases that automating can be a very time-consuming chore and can cause more work than is necessary. Look for someone who understands and knows about computers and their programming to see if what you need can be automated and if there is a program already geared to your operation.

TIPS

- *DON'T BE AFRAID OF A COMPUTER JUST BECAUSE YOU MAY BE UNFAMILIAR WITH IT. MAKE FRIENDS! IT WILL MAKE YOUR LIFE AND YOUR BUSINESS RUN SMOOTHLY!!*

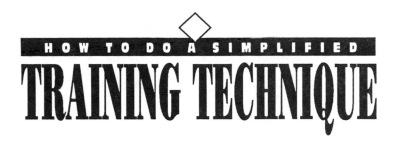

HOW TO DO A SIMPLIFIED TRAINING TECHNIQUE

It's true that time is valuable, but it will save time in the long run if your trainees get off to a good start. If you skimp on their training time, you'll pay for it later in poor work performance.

PREPARATION CHECKLIST

Make sure the people you choose to do the training are capable, efficient, and good communicators.

THE GAME PLAN

People can be trained effectively in a short amount of time. Choose a trainer with good work ethics and good work habits. Show your chosen trainer the finished product. Let the trainer know what you are hoping to achieve — the finished look, the perfect wrap, the perfect makeup, etc. Make sure the trainer knows where to get all of the necessary materials and information, then go through the training process step by step. Next, have your trainer do the work while you watch. Point out how to catch errors and correct them. Tell the trainer who can help if you are not around. Review his or her work, and allow time to practice new techniques. Above all, be available to listen if he or she has a problem.

Using someone else to coach or assist the trainee has several advantages over doing it yourself. It will save you, as the manager/owner, a lot of time and effort. The trainee may have questions that would be embarrassing to ask the boss. Trainees will acquire skills and techniques to which they might not otherwise have been exposed. After the training period, the trainee can go back to the trainer for further expertise. The process will promote closeness among your employees. You will get feedback on the progress of the trainee from the trainer.

Some people just can't learn as fast or as well as is necessary. Don't try to live with a situation where an employee cannot learn how to do the work competently. If, after a certain period of time, the trainee just can't handle the situation, then you are probably better off letting him or her go or coming to a mutual agreement about doing something else. It is unfair to the individual as well as to the owner/manager to keep that employee.

TIPS

- *REMEMBER, A GOOD TRAINING PROGRAM NOT ONLY BENEFITS YOUR BUSINESS, BUT THE EMPLOYEE WILL APPRECIATE DEVELOPING EFFICIENT SKILLS!*

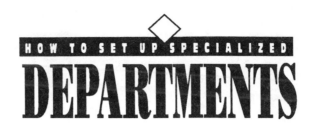

DEPARTMENTS

Like many other professions, the beauty business is getting more refined and technical every day. Just as hospitals are full of specialists, many salons now have specialized departments for perms, colors, skin care, etc.

PREPARATION CHECKLIST

Whether you are building a new salon or revamping an existing one, you need a precise plan.

THE GAME PLAN

If you are interested in specializing in your salon, it's best to start doing so at the beginning. It's very difficult to break down a salon that is already structured into specialized departments. A staff that is used to performing all services will have a tough time specializing, but it can be done. You'll probably have to let people who want to stay on the same system do so, then ask new people what their preferences would be.

A specialized department needs a department head — someone who can oversee everything. It's always good to have a person to whom the designers can go for advice.

When you specialize, you need excellent training for your people. Have systems worked out before setting up a department, and a training program in place before you hire anyone. Outline step-by-step directions for each skill you want them to learn, and have specifically designed systems so that everyone follows the same path. Teach them how to keep accurate records and to make sure that they write down all of the formulas the correct way so others can read and understand their instructions.

Each chemical department should have its own space. Have a specialist in inventory control do the ordering, separate an area for products and dispensory items, and set aside closet space for rods or color supplies.

A skin-care department should be segregated from the rest of the salon. It should have an outside entrance and be in a space separate from the salon environment. A spa should be very quiet, sedate, and serene. Keep soft music going, and have everything geared toward comfort and relaxation.

Manicures and pedicures should also have their own area. Sometimes it is uncomfortable for women to have a pedicure out in the open.

Teach your staff to promote other departments. In-house promoting is very important, especially at the desk and the cutting stations, and make sure you have enough chemical people to do the services. (An effective setup is one chemical person for every two or three designers.) A color or perm department should have a station for the client to have hair blown dry and leave if no other services are being done.

If you don't have specialized departments, every designer should be doing approximately 50 percent of total sales in haircuts and 50 percent in add-on business (chemical services).

TIPS

- *When building a new salon, check with your architect to make sure that you have all of the private rooms you will need.*
- *Make sure your receptionist knows how to book special departments so that everything runs smoothly for the client.*
- *Have separate financial statements for each department so you can compare them.*
- *SPECIALIZED DEPARTMENTS AREN'T FOR EVERYONE, BUT THEY CAN BE A REAL ASSET TO THE RIGHT BUSINESS. CONSIDER CAREFULLY WHETHER THEY'RE FOR YOU!*

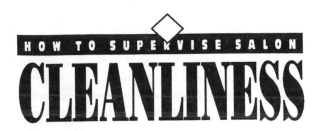

HOW TO SUPERVISE SALON
CLEANLINESS

Salon cleanliness can be the hardest thing to supervise because cleaning is basically an unrewarding job. Very few people enjoy cleaning up after someone else, but it must be done! The appearance of your shop directly affects your business. Just as you would not eat in a dirty restaurant, you cannot expect your clients to be serviced in a dirty salon.

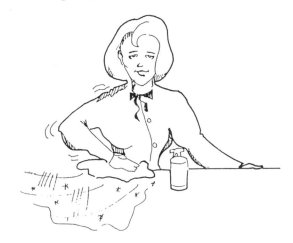

PREPARATION CHECKLIST

Unless you have a maid who is constantly cleaning and picking up after everyone, you need a system for keeping the shop neat throughout the day. Begin by making a list of things that need to be done regularly. Here are some ideas.

1. Towels laundered.
2. Floors swept.
3. Mirrors cleaned.
4. Stations cleaned.

Every employer is unique, and you will have your own ideas about what needs to be done daily in your shop.

THE GAME PLAN

Begin by assigning specific duties to specific people. This "spreads the wealth around" so no one individual feels like he or she does everything. Post a schedule of jobs, and have each person sign as he or she completes clean-up duties for the day.

Next, appoint one or two people to be floor supervisors for the month. Their job is to see that cleaning tasks get done. If the assigned person does not complete a task by the end of the day, it becomes the responsibility of the floor supervisor. It won't take long before your supervisors are making sure that all jobs are done.

Major cleaning should probably be done on a daily basis, depending upon the size of your salon. Floors should be washed, rugs swept, and windows and mirrors should be kept clean at all times. Dust products and shelves every day, and keep the front desk and reception area neat. It goes without saying that combs and brushes should be cleaned and sterilized daily, and keep your coffee area neat throughout the day.

General upkeep is also very important. Painting the walls occasionally makes the shop look a lot cleaner, and don't forget to have the rugs cleaned regularly.

Be creative with your window displays and shop decor. They should be changed periodically. Your image is formed the minute potential clients look in the salon. Make sure that what they see is what you want them to see.

Finally, take a pencil and paper and walk through your salon with your manager; write down everything that needs to be repaired, cleaned, replaced, thrown away, washed, painted, polished, or waxed. Make it a point to check places you might otherwise overlook. Then make a "to do" list, and number items in order of importance. As your budget allows, work your way through your list.

TIPS

- *When looking around, be sure to look on top of shelves and behind things. A client is sure to notice anything you have missed.*
- *When assigning jobs to your staff, change them around regularly so one person isn't stuck doing the same thing month after month.*
- *REMEMBER, A CLEAN WORKPLACE IS A POSITIVE BUSINESS IMAGE!*

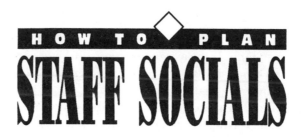

HOW TO PLAN
STAFF SOCIALS

Social events help to form strong relationships among staff members. They help the team to get to know each other socially, as well as on a business level.

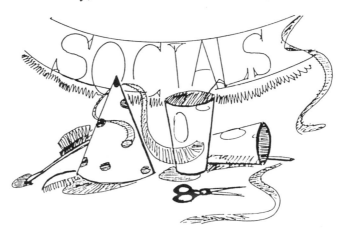

PREPARATION CHECKLIST

1. Appoint a social director to make preliminary plans.
2. Ask for a committee of volunteers to help the social director.
3. Choose a location for the event.
4. Select a date, and set up an approximate time. (It's wise to allow yourself two or three possible dates in case of a conflict.)
5. If necessary, make reservations, and, if a deposit is required, plan to collect the money in advance.
6. Make a list of supplies needed. If appropriate, you might ask each individual to bring something.
7. If it is a gift-giving occasion, decide on an amount each person should spend and what kinds of gifts are suitable.
8. If you want music, book a D.J. or band well in advance.
9. Figure out a budget for food and drinks, and plan your menu accordingly. Also consider flowers and decorations.
10. Give the occasion a dress-code: black tie, casual, etc.
11. Specify whether guests are invited. Get a head count at least two weeks before the event so you can plan the menu, seating arrangements, etc.

THE GAME PLAN

In the beginning, let everyone get involved in the planning stage. Is this going to be a Christmas party, a picnic, an awards banquet? How formal should it be, and what kind of music would they like to have? Once you have decided on the basics of the event, choose your social director and get the planning committee together. Go over their responsibilities (you might show them the PREPARATION CHECKLIST), and let them do the work.

TIPS

- *Keep your staff involved. Ask for suggestions about what kinds of things they would like to do together and how often.*
- *Try to get together socially at least four to six times a year.*
- *For a big event, such as a Christmas party, try to book your date three to four months ahead of time.*
- *For a grab bag, try having your staff members list some things they might like along with their names for a drawing. Or suggest gag gifts. They can be affordable and great fun.*
- *In planning a food budget, remember that having one or two choices for dinner can be much more cost effective than having an open menu.*
- *Dinner could be a buffet. Be sure to check the cost per plate.*
- *When serving alcohol, it is wise to limit yourself to regular mixed drinks. This will help to control your bar bill. Another way to help is to give each person a few drink tickets. (This does not include wine with dinner.) NEVER LET ANYONE DRIVE HOME AFTER DRINKING TOO MUCH.*
- *Before you decide to have a dinner in a place not already set up for it, consider the cost of renting tables, chairs, linens, china, glassware, etc. You might find that it is more expensive than the dinner itself.*
- *If you are having an awards banquet, make sure that all plaques are ordered well in advance.*
- *HAVE A WONDERFUL TIME!*

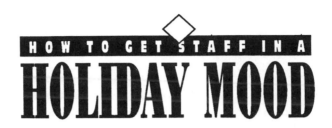

HOW TO GET STAFF IN A
HOLIDAY MOOD

Christmas is the time of year for giving, sharing, and remembering; a time to show your appreciation to your staff and your clientele.

PREPARATION CHECKLIST

1. Begin saving money in January for the next December's staff Christmas gala.
2. About two months before the holiday season, have your computer print out a list of all clients who have spent $500 or more in the salon in the last year.
3. Plan for other clients as well. (Ideas in THE GAME PLAN section.)
4. Gather a committee to decorate the salon for the holidays.

THE GAME PLAN

Christmas is a time when you should be doing everything you can to create good will among your staff and clients. You'll find it's wise to begin saving for a Christmas party in January. By December, when there are so many other expenses, a Christmas fund will allow you to have an extravaganza that you and your employees will really appreciate and enjoy. Make it a night to remember by having it at a local country club or some other nice place. Have a sit-down dinner and a gift exchange; then dance the night away!

Along with appreciating your staff, it's time to thank your clients. Suggestion: Send your VIP clients from your computer list a special Christmas message along with a four-visit card that entitles them to receive the following:

        1st visit — 20 percent discount on any chemical service

        2nd visit — 20 percent discount on any retail product

        3rd visit — free manicure with haircut

        4th visit — free gift with any service

Of course, you can make up your card any way you like.

You also do not want to forget your other clients. Consider having each member of your staff (including yourself) make several dozen cookies or candies. Purchase some small gift boxes, stuff them with the goodies, and wrap them up in holiday paper. Place them under your shop Christmas tree and hand them out to every client who comes in during the holiday week. You might also include a discount coupon in each box. Your customers will love it!

Finally, this is a good time to share with those less fortunate. Volunteer your salon's services to an old-age home, children's hospital, orphanage, etc. Pack a basket of food for a needy family, or collect toys for the poor. Make it a salon project. This is the kind of thing that makes Christmas special.

TIPS

- *If your homemade treats are really great, consider putting the recipe in the box with the goodies.*
- *HAVE A HAPPY HOLIDAY!*

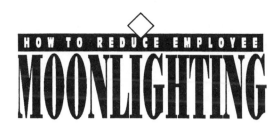

HOW TO REDUCE EMPLOYEE
MOONLIGHTING

There are few benefits to the salon from employee moonlighting.

PREPARATION CHECKLIST

Be ready to listen.

THE GAME PLAN

Employees who have second jobs are not always the most ideal workers. At times, moonlighting employees can cause the following difficulties:

1. A higher degree of absenteeism and excessive sick leave.
2. Above average tardiness.
3. Many requests to leave work early.
4. Unplanned vacation days taken sporadically.
5. Excessive fatigue during regular working hours.
6. Low availability for working extra hours.
7. Extensive breaks or lunch hours.
8. High volume of personal calls.
9. Unwillingness to accept more demanding work.

The employee's usual reason for moonlighting is needing extra income. It's a tough defense to overcome, but holding two jobs at once is not easy, and, sooner or later, the efforts can affect the regular performance. Eventually absenteeism, tardiness, and low productivity cause failure to receive raises or promotions. These problems can eventually lead to discharge.

Another drawback of moonlighting is a lack of commitment. The employee may not be as concerned about job security because of the outside income. Promotions or raises are not the significant incentives they would be. Finally, there is always the possibility that the second job will become the main job, so disciplinary measures are not really effective.

Review your company policy on moonlighting. Write down a policy that states your feelings on moonlighting. (Exceptions can be made with the approval of the manager or owner.) Make sure your employees are aware of that policy.

If there is currently someone moonlighting in your salon, and you feel that it is causing concern for your company, let the employee know how you feel. Make it clear that you don't want to lose him or her, but that he or she must decide which job is more important. Realize that there is always a possibility that you may lose the employee, but that's the chance you must take. If the manager becomes aware that a staff member is violating the moonlighting policy, he or she should face the issue immediately. A supervisor's job is much easier when employees are committed to their responsibilities and to the company.

TIPS

- *If there are alternatives for the employee, don't forget to discuss them.*
- *REMEMBER, THERE IS NO SUBSTITUTION FOR LOYALTY. FAITHFUL WORKERS ARE THE BACKBONE OF YOUR BUSINESS!*

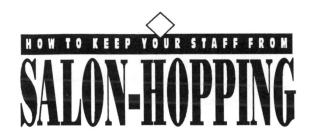

HOW TO KEEP YOUR STAFF FROM
SALON-HOPPING

Fewer young people are entering the beauty industry these days because they feel that too little money is made for all the education and effort it takes. The question is — what can be done about it? This is the time to start thinking about how we hire and educate, what benefits we offer, the management style we employ, and how we can keep the staff we have.

PREPARATION CHECKLIST

Other people in the industry will try to lure your staff away. You want to make your salon environment as pleasant as possible so your employees will want to stay. Be ready and willing to make some changes if necessary. The important thing is to be open-minded and flexible.

THE GAME PLAN

How can you protect your assets? Do a little investigating. Find out if your staff is happy with things as they are. Get their opinions. What things would they like to change, and what would make them do more or be more enthusiastic about their jobs? What ideas do they have for better staff-management relationships?

Consider hiring an outside consultant to develop a survey. Have each staff member interview privately about questions on the survey, then have the consultant write up a report telling you what things your staff wants and needs. He or she may also make some recommendations. Ask the consultant for advice on what to do about any staff members who may not be doing well.

Remember how much time and money you have invested in your employees in the first years of their employment. If they were worth hiring, it is certainly worth your while to consider their needs and desires for the future. Be willing to listen to their opinions. Keeping the lines of communication open will greatly strengthen the bonds between you and your staff, and the chances of losing them to other salons will be greatly reduced.

TIPS

- *You will help to retain the trust of your employees if you make sure to keep identities confidential in the survey questions. After all, the important thing is the result.*
- *HAVE THE MOST PLEASANT AND EXCITING SALON IN YOUR CITY AND NOT ONLY WILL YOUR EMPLOYEES STICK AROUND, BUT OTHERS WILL BE DYING TO JOIN YOU (NOT TO MENTION THE CLIENTS WHO WILL ALSO LOVE TO HANG AROUND!).*

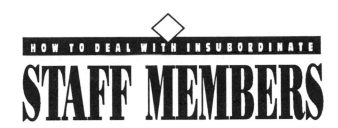

STAFF MEMBERS

Insubordination is a serious matter for both the owner/manager and for the company. A business can't survive when there is a lack of respect for authority.

PREPARATION CHECKLIST

Once again, you'll need strong self-esteem and a concrete set of standards to handle this situation.

THE GAME PLAN

Many experienced managers contend that failure to discipline a subordinate who has no valid cause for disobeying an order can lead to the following:

1. Further insubordination.
2. Declining productivity.
3. Lower employee morale.
4. Higher absenteeism and tardiness.
5. More turnover, particularly of good employees.

If an employee fails to comply with salon rules, he or she is guilty of insubordination and subject to discipline, including discharge. There are times, however, when an employee is justified in not complying with a supervisor's instructions. These might include an obvious threat to safety, contradictory instructions (a memo says to do one thing, but operators are told to do another thing), or misunderstanding instructions (however, the manager should be very explicit to people likely to misunderstand).

Any one offense cannot be punished twice. For example, if an employee is given a suspension for a week, and then, for the same incident of misconduct, is fired when he or she returns, you are liable for a lawsuit. Immediately talk to the insubordinate staff member about his or her actions and tell him or her what the possible consequences might be. Ask for an explanation of the behavior. If the explanation is not satisfactory, provide a written notice (with a copy in the employee file) stating that you have talked to him or her about a discipline problem. After two or three of these written notices, consider suspending him or her for a few days to a week. After that, you will have to consider discharge if the action continues.

TIPS

- *Discipline can be encouraged by setting good examples.*
- *ALWAYS BE WILLING TO LISTEN TO AN EMPLOYEE BEFORE TAKING ANY ACTION. YOU MAY SAVE YOURSELF SOME AGGRAVATION, AND YOU'LL BE PROTECTING YOUR INTERESTS AS WELL!*

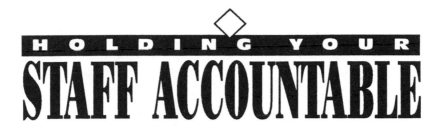

HOLDING YOUR STAFF ACCOUNTABLE

Sometimes a leader or coach has to be tough-minded when it comes to getting results from your staff. You cannot tolerate excuses when attainable goals are not being met.

PREPARATION CHECKLIST

Be sure to have all of the facts before you accuse someone of an offense or blame a person for some situation.

THE GAME PLAN

When the deficiency is first noticed, acknowledge it and approach the individual. Try to find out what the problems are. Don't allow anyone to blame someone else or circumstances for something that is clearly his or her problem. Your staff should know that when they accept their jobs, they are accountable for their actions.

After you have all of the facts, listen to each side of the story. If this doesn't take care of the problem, let the parties involved know how you feel. Give them a certain amount of time to correct the situation, and state the consequences if it is not resolved. Let them know you care about them and the situation, but that certain things cannot be tolerated. Then stand your ground.

Suggestions for consequences: After a verbal warning, write the employee a letter, a copy of which should be kept in the employee file. It should detail performance deficiencies and outline the expected results during the next week or month. Include everything that was discussed with the individual. If the letter does not stimulate improvement, the next step should be time off without pay. Advise the offender to spend the time thinking about the seriousness of the offense. Of course, the final step would be dismissal.

TIPS

- *Never give a warning letter without first speaking to the individual.*
- *Never say anything negative about the employee. Address only the action with which you don't agree.*
- *REMEMBER, IF YOU IGNORE SUBSTANDARD WORK, IT WILL BECOME THE NORMAL OR ACCEPTABLE WAY OF OPERATING.*

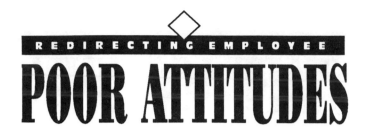

REDIRECTING EMPLOYEE
POOR ATTITUDES

The most difficult problem to deal with is poor attitude. This problem is not as obvious, but is as damaging to your business as others.

PREPARATION CHECKLIST

Make sure that this is the problem with which you are dealing and see if you can discover a cause.

THE GAME PLAN

These are some of the traits of a poor attitude.

1. Low productivity unless under direct pressure.
2. Low quality work (and not taking responsibility for errors).
3. Distrust of supervisors and managers.
4. Antagonism towards the company and its management.
5. Disregarding instructions.
6. Slow compliance with changes in work methods.
7. Quickly pointing out any drawbacks of any new system initiated.
8. Seldom volunteering to do any extra work.
9. Largely uncooperative with conscientious employees.

The employee with a poor attitude usually keeps a low profile, not talking much and keeping thoughts and opinions to him- or herself. He or she vents true feelings in a more subtle way. It is not likely to be an outright act of defiance, because he or she doesn't want to get caught.

For the long term, be sure that all instructions given to this employee are clear and precise. Leave no doubt about what should be accomplished. Set time limits for completion of jobs. Instruct other staff members to let you know if work is roadblocked. Reinforce all self-checking procedures and the required standards for all work. Be sure the employee understands when and how to coordinate work with others. Check his or her progress regularly. After a couple of weeks of implementing this "careful eye" approach, let up a little. See if you have a reversal in work habits. The employee may overcome minor problems in his or her work and develop a willingness to do extra work. He or she may become more cooperative with other workers and make fewer errors. You may hear fewer negative comments. If this is the case you have successfully turned the problem around. If not, you may need to communicate that overall attitude needs improvement and that you want to see a change in the way that he or she approaches the work. Give him or her a time period in which to work on improving attitude. You may see a change. If not, give him or her a warning and, after three written warnings, you may be forced to dismiss the employee.

TIPS

- *As with any other discipline problem, listen to your employee first. Perhaps something is causing the problem that can be resolved easily.*
- *DON'T IGNORE A POOR ATTITUDE. CORRECTING IT WILL HELP THE EMPLOYEE AT WORK AND AT HOME AND WILL BOOST THE MORALE OF OTHER EMPLOYEES!*

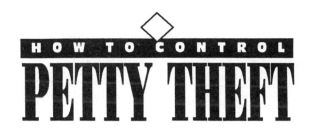

HOW TO CONTROL PETTY THEFT

Few matters can be as vexing as suspecting that a worker is a thief. Whether it is company property or that of other employees, it must be stopped.

PREPARATION CHECKLIST

Gather all facts before accusing any person.

THE GAME PLAN

Stealing, no matter what the value of the property, has to be viewed with alarm. One must suppose that if a culprit is caught with a minor item, he or she might have an inclination to do worse. The disappearance of small items can eventually lead to more valuable items such as pocketbooks, wallets, tools, personal items, money, etc. Here is a checklist to help curb theft:

1. Put things away. Use desk drawers, closets, file cabinets, and money drawers with locks. This will reduce temptation and availability.
2. Allow one person to be in charge of collecting money for the desk, or have the receptionist account for the day's receipts.
3. Keep large amounts of materials and products in a restricted and locked area. Put as little of a product as is needed for a day in the dispensary.
4. Advise employees that they are responsible for their own property and that there is no company reimbursement for their losses.
5. Have a policies and procedures manual relating to stealing and theft. State what the consequences will be if anyone is caught.
6. If someone else is responsible for ordering, make sure you check the inventory or work list prior to placing an order and after its arrival. Look for any quantities above the normal products and amounts that you need.
7. Never confront an employee on the basis of circumstantial evidence.
8. Compliance with security procedures should be extremely tight for any employee about whom the supervisor is suspicious.

TIPS

- *WHEN CONDUCTING AN INVESTIGATION INTO THEFT, BE VERY THOROUGH AND ALWAYS BE WILLING TO LISTEN TO AN EXPLANATION .*

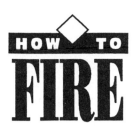

HOW TO FIRE

Running a business has its good and bad moments, but anyone who has had to fire someone will tell you that this is probably one of the most stressful things you will encounter. Although we never start out thinking we'll have to do it, situations arise when the decision must be made.

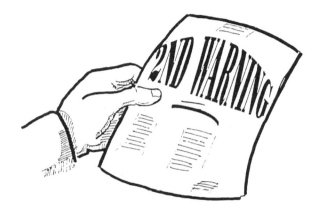

PREPARATION CHECKLIST

Keep a written file on all offenses. Assemble the facts, including dates and times, to document your case. Some possible reasons for dismissal are the following:

1. Poor attendance.
2. Constantly arriving late and/or leaving early.
3. Poor attitude towards co-workers and clients.
4. Low productivity levels.
5. Insubordination.
6. Drug and alcohol offenses.
7. Theft.
8. Other evidence of misconduct.

THE GAME PLAN

Before you fire someone, you should issue at least three warnings. The first could be verbal; the second and third should be written and signed by the employee. He or she should be warned of the consequences of continued misconduct. After three warnings you can safely dismiss the employee without legal consequences, if your reasons have been sufficiently documented.

You should try to encourage voluntary resignation, if possible. Some of the typical inducements are:

1. Letting the employee know that his or her performance is unsatisfactory.
2. Minimizing salary increases (percentage is decreased) or stopping them altogether.
3. Reducing promotions.
4. Scheduling inconvenient working hours.
5. Assigning tedious duties.
6. Constantly monitoring time and work.
7. Booking fewer clients.

TIPS

- *Give the employee every possible opportunity before making your decision. Take time and effort to look into each matter individually prior to your final decision.*
- *REMEMBER, SOMETIMES AN INDIVIDUAL MUST BE FIRED FOR THE GOOD OF THE BUSINESS. TRUST YOURSELF ON THIS ONE.*

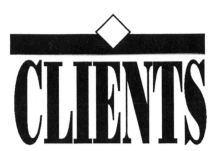

CLIENTS

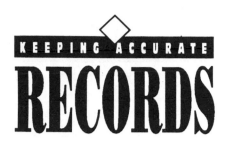

KEEPING ACCURATE RECORDS

One of the most important things in your business is to keep accurate records. You must update data constantly. Without proper records, it is very difficult to run your business.

PREPARATION CHECKLIST

Be prepared to get organized!

THE GAME PLAN

If you have a computer, you are fortunate. If not, have your clients fill out customer cards with all of the data that you'll need for promotions: full name, address, occupation, sex, family information. This information will help you determine the type of salon you run. It will also help with marketing and promotions.

It is equally important to keep proper records of each client's services. With exact formulas written down, you're less likely to make perm or color mistakes — and if you do, you'll never repeat them! Furthermore, if a particular designer is sick, another designer will be able to look at the client's card and perform the proper service for that client. The customer's needs must always come first.

Many reports and systems can be used in a beauty salon. If your business is computerized, you can run productivity reports that will show you how many chemicals, haircuts, and conditioners each person sold. If not, you'll need to assemble this information yourself. Computer reports are also valuable when it is time to evaluate your staff. You can't accurately give a good evaluation if you don't know the facts. Data must be updated regularly so you know who has changed names or moved, etc. This will keep you from wasting time and money mailing to incorrect names and/or addresses. Generally, this is part of the front desk person's job. If you work alone, keeping records will be even more difficult if you are not computerized. You must keep track of the most important things — client cards, formula cards, addresses, and phone numbers. It's also good to know what products you purchased so you can fill the need next time.

TIPS

- *Formulate a card for each type of information you require and then color code or put tabs on them. It will help you to be organized.*
- *IF YOU DO NOT ALREADY HAVE ONE, THINK SERIOUSLY ABOUT GETTING A COMPUTER. IT WILL SAVE YOU TIME AND MONEY. IT'S THE WAY OF THE 90S!*

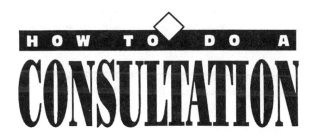

HOW TO DO A
CONSULTATION

A consultation is probably the most important first step toward achieving a happy client. When you take the time to learn about a person, it is easier to suggest a suitable look that matches the personality. Clients are more comfortable when they feel that you understand them. They are more likely to trust your advice because you really care about them.

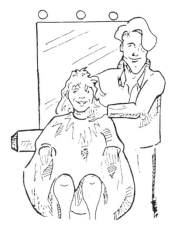

PREPARATION CHECKLIST

1. Set aside enough time. Don't try to rush a consultation.
2. Have a list of questions ready or a form prepared that will help you get to know your potential client.
3. No matter what kind of day you are having, smile. You only get one chance to make a first impression!

THE GAME PLAN

Shake hands with your new client (a firm handshake speaks wonders to a new friend!) and thank him or her for coming to your salon. Ask the client how he or she heard about you (this is helpful information; it tells you what advertising methods are working). Make it clear that you appreciate his or her business.

Next, sit down with your client, face to face. Don't look through a mirror. Observe the client's clothes and hairstyle. Is it conservative, sporty, professional, fun? Try to understand the client's needs. If you see some major mistakes (or if the client feels someone has made a mistake) offer to correct the situation, but never say anything negative about another person's work. It's not professional.

Ask questions in a conversational tone so your client will feel comfortable, but remember that time is money. You want to gather as much information as you can in the time set aside. Find out about lifestyle. How much time does the client spend on hair, and what products does he or she use? Finally, does the client have a picture of what he or she is trying to achieve?

TIPS

- *Always LISTEN to your client. Don't be thinking about what you will say next while your client is talking.*
- *Don't promise something you can't deliver. You'll always lose in the end. Be honest. If the client has thin, straight, baby-fine hair and wants a look with a lot of curl and volume, explain why it can't be done, and suggest something else. (This is where your observations come in.) If his or her hair is not in condition to achieve a specific perm, color, or cut, don't attempt it. Advise the client to condition it before you can perform the service.*
- *Don't treat people differently. Treat each client as if he or she is your first client on your first day.*
- *Don't pressure someone into getting a service he or she doesn't want. Again, you'll be the loser.*
- *Never cut more hair than you said you would even if you think it will look better. You could have a very unhappy, former client.*
- *MAKE A GOOD IMPRESSION, AND YOU WILL HAVE A NEW FRIEND AS WELL AS A FAITHFUL CLIENT!*

SAMPLE CONSULTATION SHEET

Facial shape: _____

   Problems: _____

   Corrections: _____

Profile: _____

   Problems: _____

   Corrections: _____

Personality: _____

Lifestyle: _____

Profession: _____

Texture: _____

Density: _____

Perm: _____

Hair color: _____

Hair products: _____

Upkeep: _____

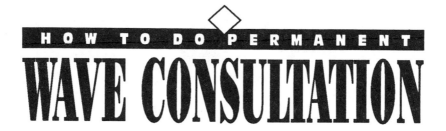

WAVE CONSULTATION

Determining your client's needs and desires before perming his or her hair will insure you of having a happy, satisfied customer.

PREPARATION CHECKLIST

1. You will need a general information sheet for your client to fill out.
2. Prepare either a perm questionnaire for her to answer or a list of questions for you to ask during your consultation.

THE GAME PLAN

As hair designers, we know that it's important to know the answers to a number of questions before exposing a client's hair to chemical processes. If you have booked a perm for a brand new client, fill out the general information sheet (see "How to Do a Consultation") first. After that, for new and old clients, complete a questionnaire that deals specifically with permanent waving, or at least ask the questions. Here are some of the questions you will need to ask.

1. How long has it been since your last perm?
2. Have you ever experienced an allergic reaction to perm solution?
3. What length was your hair at the time of your last perm? Is it the same length now? What were the results?
4. What kind of curl pattern are you looking for — tight, medium, or loose?
5. What method of styling will you be using on your hair — setting or blow drying?
6. What products do you use on your hair?
7. Can you handle your hair easily? Are you willing and able to take care of a time-consuming style?
8. What profession are you in? (This determines an appropriate look. Ask the client to show you a picture of what he or she has in mind.)

After you have answered the questions, be honest with your client. Don't say you can do something if it is not possible. You'll gain the client's confidence by telling the truth.

TIPS

- *If a client's hair is too damaged to perm, let him or her know that you will do all you can to restore it so you can do a perm at a future date.*

77

- *Don't tell a client with weak, fine, thin hair that you can create a style with lots of volume. If the client can't accept the truth, you're better off losing him or her than taking the chance of ruining the hair and having the client tell others what a horrible job you do.*

- *BE HONEST AND REALISTIC AS WELL AS CREATIVE, AND THE MAJORITY OF YOUR CLIENTS WILL NOT ONLY APPRECIATE YOU, BUT WILL SPREAD THE WORD!*

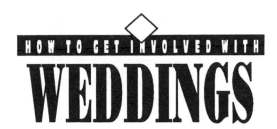

HOW TO GET INVOLVED WITH
WEDDINGS

The wedding industry is a very large business and can bring a lot of money into your salon. It's nice to put services together for brides and their families before their weddings and to give them a package for their special day as well.

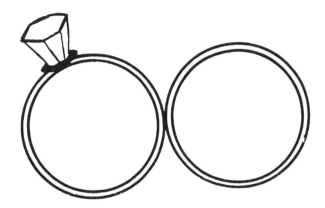

PREPARATION CHECKLIST

1. Be ready to discuss and show different hairstyles to the bride. Have pictures there to show her some suggestions.
2. Set aside enough time so the bride does not feel rushed.

THE GAME PLAN

You can get involved in many ways. Look for a bridal fair or bridal show in your area and find out who runs it. (Call your local bridal stores — they can usually tell you.) Ask them if you could do hair for such a show. Ask if they have booths and, if so, could you purchase a booth and hand out literature or show some of your work? It's also good to hand out coupons or another incentive to make people want to come for a consultation. Try to get them to sign their names and addresses to a guest list. This gives you data for a mailing list of potential brides. Sometimes the host organization will give you a mailing list for your participation in the show. Then you can send mailings (see chapter entitled "How to Do Direct Mailings") to brides.

Have a couple of different packages put together. One might be just for the bride and another for her entire bridal party, or package a visit for a trial run and one for the wedding day itself for a certain price. Maybe you will want to include manicures and makeup in that price; or try a home package. Contact bridal agencies or stores to see if you can cross-promote within each other's places of business. Exchange business cards. This is a good reference. And don't forget to promote to your existing clientele as well as at bridal fairs. You might even suggest that you will go with the bridal party to the photographer if they have scheduled a shoot prior to the wedding.

TIPS

- *Why not include the groom and/or groomsmen in a package? Maybe you could offer a free or discounted haircut to the men earlier in the month when the bridal party agrees to come in for the wedding day.*
- *THIS KIND OF BUSINESS GIVES YOU AN OPPORTUNITY TO BE CREATIVE AND TO SPREAD A LOT OF JOY AS WELL!*

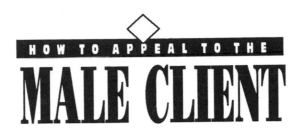

HOW TO APPEAL TO THE
MALE CLIENT

In the recent past, more and more men have switched from barbers to hair salons, and a lot of places now service a large male clientele. Men are a relatively new source of income for the modern salon, and it's important that you make them comfortable without losing your appeal to women.

PREPARATION CHECKLIST

Unless your salon is frilly and feminine, the changes you might want to make shouldn't be too hard. Put yourself in a man's place, and imagine how he might feel coming to your salon, then plan your changes accordingly.

THE GAME PLAN

Some of those changes might be:

1. Your salon should be generic. When planning your decor, use neutral colors.
2. Make sure your promotions and advertising are geared toward anyone. Incorporate men in your ads, and promote within your salon for the male by asking your female clients to bring in husbands, sons, and friends.
3. Do makeovers for males and females.

It's easy to promote to males, and usually they are excellent customers. Businessmen will get their hair cut every three weeks, so they are a great source of fill-in business. Men also have a lot of color and perms done, but you want to do these things subtly. Men generally don't want it to be too noticeable, whereas a woman might be less concerned. For example, a man might want just a little color brushed on to take away the grey look in his sideburns.

Make your male client comfortable. Don't give him a flowered smock. Make sure you have magazines in the waiting area geared toward his interests, like *Business Times* or *Newsweek*. Most men don't like to wait long, especially businessmen, so have a system where you can call them if the stylist is running late; or ask them to call in to see how you are running. Plan your time schedule accordingly. Try doing a promotion to encourage them to come in at lunch hour, but make sure your designer is able to get them in and out on time.

Gear the style to the individual, and try not to create a look he doesn't like. Notice the type of job he has or how he dresses when he comes in, and that will help you determine the cut. Always ask him to take off his shirt and tie and put on a smock so he doesn't have hair on his neck for the rest of the day. If he chooses not to wear a smock, make sure you cover his shirt collar with a towel to keep him from getting itchy when he goes back to work. Always remove the hair from his ears and trim his eyebrows. These are extra services that men really enjoy.

TIPS

- *Plan a Father's Day special — "Two for One ** Bring Your Mate!"*
- *MEN BRING IN NEW BUSINESS, AND THEY'RE GREAT TO BE AROUND! ENCOURAGE YOUR STYLISTS TO ENCOURAGE THEM!*

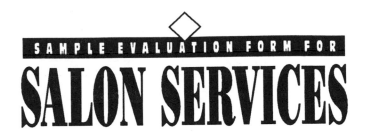

SAMPLE EVALUATION FORM FOR
SALON SERVICES

There is nothing more important than feedback for your business. The more you know about your clients' feelings and expectations, the easier it will be to address their needs. Every hotel and restaurant asks you to fill out a survey sheet. It shows how they can better serve you. Why not do that in our salons?

PREPARATION CHECKLIST

You are preparing to develop a survey concerning the services in your salon. Consider every aspect that affects the client. Walk around your shop and take notes. Look for everything and anything that might affect a customer.

THE GAME PLAN

The following is a sample survey. You can use it as is, add to or subtract from it, or change it to suit your particular shop.

Client's Name _____

Address _____

City or Town _____ Sex _____

Marital Status _____ Occupation _____

How far from (name of salon) do you live? _____

Age Range _____ Birthday _____

Please rate the indicated questions from 1 to 5.
1: Poor   2: Fair   3: Good   4: Very Good   5: Outstanding

1. Was this your first visit to (name of salon)? .... ☐ Yes ☐ No
2. How would you rate your overall experience at (name of salon)?
  ....1 2 3 4 5
3. Were you treated courteously on the telephone? 1 2 3 4 5
4. How would you rate your designer's work? 1 2 3 4 5
5. Do you feel that we achieved the look you wanted? .... ☐ Yes ☐ No

6. What, to you, is the most important aspect of your visit to a professional salon?
   _____
   _____

7. Were you kept waiting too long? .... ☐ Yes ☐ No
8. Were any of our professional products recommended to you? ☐ Yes ☐ No
   Did you purchase any? .... ☐ Yes ☐ No
   If yes, do you have any comments to make? _____
   _____

9. Who was your designer? _____
   What did you like about her/him? _____
   _____
   Is there anything that she/he could have improved? _____
   _____

10. Is there anything else we could have done to make your experience more
    satisfying and enjoyable? _____
    _____

11. Will you be visiting us again? .... ☐ Yes ☐ No
    If not, why not? _____
12. Please indicate which of the following services you use or might be interested in
    using. Perms, haircuts, facials, etc. (List services you use and those that you
    might like to start.) _____
    _____

13. Would you be more likely to use one or more of these services if they were
    available at one salon? .... ☐ Yes ☐ No
14. May we ask the name of the salon you currently use or have used in the past?
    _____

15. May we put you on our mailing list for future specials, promotions, and our
    newsletter? .... ☐ Yes ☐ No
16. Do you have a friend or relative for whom we could provide a complementary
    consultation or haircut?
    Name_____ Telephone # _____

Thank you so much for your time and help in completing this evaluation. We thank you
again for visiting our salon; it was a pleasure having you as our guest.

TIPS

- *For taking the time to fill out the questionnaire, consider giving your client a small
  sample gift or a percentage off of his or her next visit.*
- *Don't forget to use the information obtained in your survey to evaluate your staff
  and in your marketing plan.*
- *THIS IS YOUR CUSTOMER SERVICE GAUGE. USE IT TO BECOME THE
  BEST SALON IN TOWN!*

PERSONAL DEVELOPMENT

Born in England, Raised in the US. Professional Career has included working near the Chagrin Blvd area in top salons, JoJo A Salon on Oak St. in Chicago, and the Jean-Louis - David Salon at Henri Bendels in N.Y.C.

work of Ann's family + loved ones are in Cleveland and so she purchased Larderwood Hair Kansas in 1996 and have renovated and updated the spot to Larderwood Hair & Spa, a full service salon + spa including hair, nails, facials, massage. waxing, treatments

Ann's other passions are music (she is a cantor at St. Noel's Church in W. Hills), sailing, and horse back riding).

Ann has been seen doing hair on the Morning Exchange, and is a working owner, four day busy working being the professional styling chair Wed - Sat. An advocate of advanced education. She constantly is keeping her work current by attending up with trends classes in L.A. and N.Y.

Ann believes that a woman needs to develop her own personal style., choosing one that not only compliments her face + hair texture, but lifestyle also. She feels strongly about adapting that special look or style to the clients facial features, head shape, posture, hair texture, + ease of care. She feels life is complicated enough · your hair should be easy + fun

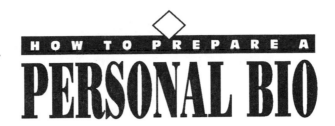

HOW TO PREPARE A
PERSONAL BIO

Your biographies, or "bios," are used for all kinds of marketing and promotional campaigns that you might do for your business. It's important that you have a bio prepared in case you would like to do something outside of the salon. You can send a photograph and your bio to manufacturers if you are looking for a promotion or a job or you can send your bio with a picture to a newspaper for a press release. There are many possibilities.

PREPARATION CHECKLIST

The first thing that you need to do is to collect some data. Here are some of the things you might include.

1. Family history, marital status, address, number of children.
2. All history or scrapbook items you have saved from your career.
3. All trophies, awards, accomplishments, and recognitions you may have received during your time in the industry.
4. Any organizations, manufacturers, or groups for which you may have worked or of which you are a member.
5. List your outstanding characteristics, hobbies, outside activities, and/or charity organizations with which you deal.
6. Articles you may have published, magazines with your photos or work.
7. Your personal philosophy and your philosophy about our industry.
8. Whether or not you have ownership in a business, or the title of your job and its description.
9. Your strongest talents and things of which you are most proud.
10. Educational background, including advanced education.

THE GAME PLAN

Once you have collected all of this data, highlight all of the things you feel are most important and then give it to a writer who can help you put your bio together; or write it yourself if you are talented in this area. Sometimes it's easier, however, to have someone else write about you than to write about yourself. It is important to have two different bios for different situations. You need a brief one (a couple of lines or so) for perhaps a newspaper story, as well as a more extensive one that you might use in a resume, for example. Try to get

⟹ but you must be realistic to do this. ~~this is very~~

"color should compliment the cut. Cut 1st. Color 2nd. Skin care

87

all of your information on one page so there is no likelihood of a page being lost or separated. Have your bio typeset and copied by a printer so it looks professional.

TIPS

- *Don't use lengthy, complicated sentences. Be concise, and make your bio easy to read and understand.*
- *YOU'RE SELLING YOURSELF HERE, SO DON'T HESITATE TO HIGHLIGHT ALL OF YOUR STRONG POINTS!*

is often overlooked. European women have been taking care of their skin for years. Americans tend to neglect then go straight to the surgeon's cutting table - plastic surgeons. Too many of these women look like they have had "work done."

"Eyes are the focal point of the face" I understand, see an eye lift bluntly? when it is necessary, but there are alternatives to the face lift. Regular facial massage helps keep the facial muscles toned and now we have micro-dermabrasion to light to medium exfoliation. Most clients require 4 to 8 treatments to help with fine lines, eradicate scars, dark pigmentation, and even active acne. It is progressive procedure, not aggressive, with the top layer of the skin.

There are other uses for m.D. also. It may also be used on the body to alleviate stretch marks, smooth the skin on neck, chest, & decolatte areas. Even brown spots on the hands.

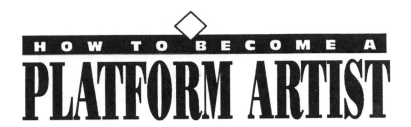

HOW TO BECOME A
PLATFORM ARTIST

Many stylists would like to grow beyond just working on clients. If you have good technical and speaking skills, you might want to consider working with a manufacturer or distributor as a platform artist.

PREPARATION CHECKLIST

Find out who your local distributors are and when they will be having shows or educationals. If you are well qualified to teach and do platform work, make a list of the manufacturers for whom you might want to work.

THE GAME PLAN

To start out, volunteer your services to local distributors for any shows they might be doing. You will usually find that they need help in the back room shampooing, organizing, finding models, etc. Plan not to be paid the first time. There is a better chance that they will agree this way. Leave a bio or resume with the distributor or show coordinator. Tell this person what interests you and what services you can provide. If you have a portfolio, bring it along. If not, plan to do some sessions so your work can be seen.

If you would like to do platform work, send your bio, a summary of your experience, photos of your work, and a cover letter to manufacturers on your list. Apply for a "salon tech" position. This position requires you to go to salons and do educationals featuring the manufacturer's products. Usually this leads to doing larger shows and educationals.

TIPS

- *Without question, your teaching, speaking, and people skills should be excellent. Get involved in the industry. Find yourself a mentor or someone who can guide you. Get to know the people who make things happen.*
- *PEOPLE WHO ARE ON STAGE HAD TO DO SOMETHING TO GET THERE. REMEMBER, YOU HAVE TO PUT IN THE TIME AND EFFORT TO REAP THE BENEFITS.*

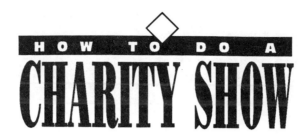

CHARITY SHOW

A charity show is a great way to give to and help out less fortunate people. It can also be an opportunity to expose your work to a lot of people who otherwise might not be aware of it.

PREPARATION CHECKLIST

1. Choose the charity, either with your staff or on your own, with which you would like to work.
2. Contact the person in charge of the designated charity.
3. Set up a meeting with all of the decision-makers.
4. Outline what you would like to do for the charity.
5. If possible, list all the expenses you're likely to have and the projected amount you could bring in as revenue.
6. Write a proposal of what your responsibilities will be and what the charity will do.
7. Draw up a budget.

THE GAME PLAN

Begin by breaking down the event into different committees; for example, the decorating committee, the food committee, invitations, etc. Then pick a chairperson with strong leadership and organizational skills. Also choose an honorary chairperson who can draw an audience with his or her presence. This person should be a television, radio, or community celebrity.

Next, look for corporations who will donate money to sponsor the event. Also look for other kinds of donations like flowers, decorations, gifts or prizes, or services such as hairdressers, makeup artists, printers, etc. Make sure you know how much the charitable organization itself will help in the project, and check the budget to see if you can get any financial help for expenses along the way.

Try to get an advertising or promotions person to market it for you. The more exposure you get the more successful it will be, and, if it is a show, assign someone to be the producer. You will need someone in charge to make all the final decisions and to keep things organized.

Choose a facility in which to hold your event that is capable of holding the number of people you expect. Make sure the room has the capacity for the staging, lighting, etc. that you will need. Consider accommodations that already have these capabilities, as they are very costly to rent. Find out whether or not the place is unionized. This also can be expensive, as you will be required to follow union rules.

What foods will your budget allow? A sit-down dinner is much more expensive than finger foods or desserts. And how much will you charge to attend? Make sure you target your audience. Ticket pricing can determine the number of people you want.

Finally, and perhaps most important, after you have decided what you want done and who you want to do it, set up a time schedule. It is imperative that in a project of this magnitude everyone works together and things get done on time.

TIPS

- *Allow six months to one year to plan for the event. Adequate time can make all the difference in the world in the quality of the outcome.*
- *Choose committee members who are organized, dependable, and have the time to devote to the cause.*
- *List all of the expenses that need to be covered and, when money is distributed, make sure all lines of communications are open between all the committees so that no misunderstandings occur.*
- *RAISE LOTS OF MONEY, BE A BENEFIT TO THE COMMUNITY, AND GET YOUR NAME AND WORK KNOWN.*

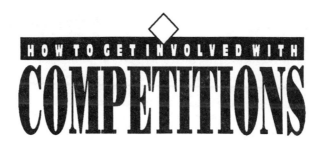

HOW TO GET INVOLVED WITH COMPETITIONS

You were probably exposed to competitions early in your beauty school days. Most schools run competitions for fun and excitement or as a project for creativity, and they can continue to be exciting far beyond beauty school!

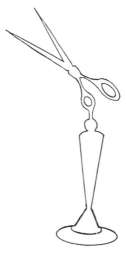

PREPARATION CHECKLIST

Do you have the time, patience, desire, and ability?

THE GAME PLAN

There are many things that you must know about competing in order to be successful at it. Probably the most important thing is finding the correct model. Find the best face, a nice body, and the right kind of hair for the competition in which you are entering. Look at the hairline, the facial structure, the texture, etc. and make sure that the look you are trying to create will be very good on this particular face. The face is more important than anything else. If you have a nice face and a nice overall appearance, the judges will notice that first.

When you enter a competition, it's important that you understand the rules and regulations. Read them carefully, including the "fine print." Understand all the little guidelines. Be very well prepared and practice a number of times for the look that you are tying to create. Make sure the color of the hair that you are working on is perfected. If it is a color competition, practice it a couple of times to be sure that it will look right. Remember, competition is judged on its accuracy. When you haven't practiced enough, you risk looking very bad in the eyes of your peers.

Once you've started entering national or international competitions, it's time to consider hiring a trainer. Because of the intricacies involved, a trainer can guide you through all of the necessary requirements. If you are truly interested, there are many people available who can help you. Contact the National Hairdresser's Association or any group involved in competition for further information.

Another important thing to consider about competition is wardrobe. How is your model going to be dressed? Be sure that the outfit matches the hairstyle and completes the look from head to toe. If it's an evening competition, don't dress your model in jeans. If it's a makeup or nail competition, the judging staff may require something specific. Be sure to follow the guidelines.

In conclusion, the most important thing to stress is PRACTICE. Nothing that you do in competition will be successful without it. Be completely familiar with the overall look you are trying to achieve, and you will do very well.

TIPS

- *Don't ever go into a competition unprepared.*
- *If you don't have the time and the patience to put into this, don't get involved.*
- *FORMULA FOR SUCCESS: PRACTICE, PRACTICE, PRACTICE!!!*

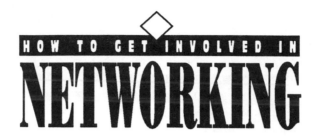

NETWORKING

Networking is very important to our personal and business growth. It's something that we should all consider if we are in business or if we're working in a business that requires us to acquire a clientele.

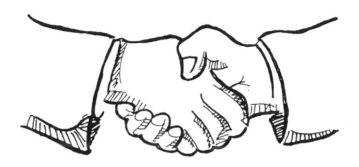

PREPARATION CHECKLIST

Find out what sort of business and social associations are available in your area.

THE GAME PLAN

The following are a few of the places to begin to build a good network: any local charity functions; anything to do with community affairs, bazaars, street fairs, etc.; associations for women in business; Toastmaster's groups; the Dale Carnegie groups; consulting companies; private business partners; the National Hairdresser's Association (NHDA); all local distributor hair shows; night club shows and functions; volunteer groups; investment groups; business conventions; anything to do with your favorite hobbies; golf clubs, country clubs, etc. Networking with some of these associations can help you with your business or help you promote some of your own clientele. It's important to get involved in your community, and it's worth all of the effort you put into it. People will begin to recognize you as a leader in your profession. They will want to use your services because you are a giver.

Get involved with a church group doing volunteer work, or go to a school, volunteer, and network with the teachers and parents. You might network in some parents' associations to

94

build part of your business from those people. Most importantly, share and learn new ideas and skills from others. Finding a mentor or someone who you feel is very good in what you would like to learn is something that you can't just buy. Finding someone who can help you do what you want to do is probably one of the best things you can do to be successful.

TIPS

- *Be sincere. Don't let people think you are just using them to drum up business. LET THEM KNOW YOU REALLY CARE ABOUT WHATEVER YOU ARE DOING.*

GETTING INVOLVED WITH A
DISTRIBUTOR-SALES REP

Many people in our industry are not comfortable working behind a chair and would like to do other things. One of those options might be working with a distributor as a salesperson.

PREPARATION CHECKLIST

Are you a good "talker"? Do you have a desire to sell, and are you dissatisfied with the traditional salon setting? This is an area to consider.

THE GAME PLAN

A sales rep might visit a salon to introduce a product, teach a class, or help with inventory control. He or she might show a salon owner how to put an inventory control system together. With your understanding and knowledge of the industry, you have a definite advantage over the layperson.

Many opportunities can be found with manufacturers and distributors. You can work for a manufacturer and distribute products throughout a salon or an area, or you can work through a distributor and help sell his or her products.

Along with selling products, distributors and manufacturers put on exhibitions in different areas or sometimes get involved with national shows. The salesperson may be responsible for helping put these shows together, and/or putting bag deals or promotions together for salon owners and designers to purchase products at the show for a discounted price. These shows can be on a local, national, or international level. A lot of work and detail goes into planning one of these shows, presenting varied opportunities for growth and creativity.

Distributors are not just order takers. You don't want to be someone who walks in and says, "What do you want today?" You want to be able to help people and help salons with any problems that they might have concerning inventory, retailing, sales training, or product knowledge. Offering suggestions and spending time with these people can greatly benefit you as well as your company.

TIPS

- *Know your product line. Make sure you'll be able to answer any questions that might come up.*

- *Believe in your product. It's hard to sell something in which you don't have confidence.*
- *ALWAYS BE FAIR WITH YOUR CLIENTS. THIS WILL ENHANCE YOUR REPUTATION AND YOUR BUSINESS, AND IT MAY BRING NEW FRIENDS INTO YOUR LIFE!!*

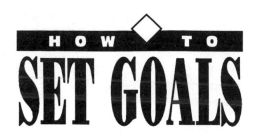

SET GOALS

Life is full of decisions. Some of us welcome decisions with excitement and anticipation, while others look for ways to avoid them. The latter are only fooling themselves, because a decision avoided is a decision to do nothing. Most people spend so much time trying not to fail that they never get around to being successful. It's easier to stay where you are than to venture into something new.

Centuries ago, Socrates advised his students, "Know thyself." His advice is still valid today. If your life is to have meaning, you must have a purpose, and, to have a purpose, you must have goals.

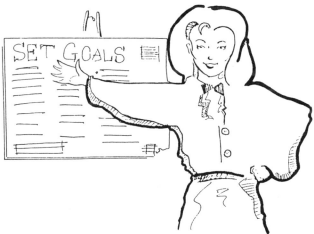

PREPARATION CHECKLIST

1. An open, inquiring mind.
2. A good attitude.
3. Creative visualization skills.
4. Pen and paper.
5. A quiet and peaceful place to think.
6. A commitment to success.

THE GAME PLAN

In the next eight topics, we are going to explore specific areas of goal-setting. We will explore how to focus your mind in every aspect of your life — think it through thoroughly and set worthwhile goals, realistic and attainable.

Once you develop ideas, write them down. Then try to list them in some kind of priority, with those most important to you on top. When you've done that in each category, summarize ten of your top choices, devise a plan, and begin to work on them.

TIPS

- *Give yourself a time frame in which to work — a limit that will give you a realistic opportunity to achieve your aim. If your list is too long, you might lose your focus and become lazy and discouraged, but if it is too short, you will become frustrated and will be setting yourself up for failure. Try beginning with a year. Some goals will be met long before that time, and others may need more time, but it's a good starting point.*

- *Don't lock yourself into the above time frame too tightly. If you reach your goal early, fantastic! But, if you find that you need more time, don't get discouraged. Circumstances can change unexpectedly, so be flexible — because life is!*

- *Make your goals realistic. Seeing yourself as an instant millionaire when you work as a waitress in a fast food store sets you up for disappointment. The facts are you can never make a million dollars working as a waitress ... but you can as the owner of a restaurant!*

- *LEARN TO VISUALIZE YOUR GOALS. IF YOU CAN SEE IT, YOU CAN MAKE IT HAPPEN!*

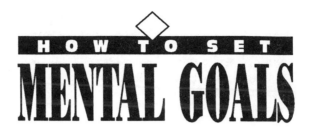

HOW TO SET
MENTAL GOALS

Mental goals deal with how you think, how you visualize, and what you want your self-image to be.

PREPARATION CHECKLIST

1. Have paper and pen.
2. Be ready to think ...

THE GAME PLAN

Take your pen and paper into a quiet place and begin to think about your general long-term goals. Where do you want to be in ten years or so? Then begin to narrow it down. How are you going to get there in terms of mental short-term goals? Are you the type of person who believes in him- or herself, or do you need to work on your self-esteem? What kind of an education do you have, and what further training do you need? What kinds of self-improvement studies do you want to pursue? Consider recreational and professional areas, personal development, speed-reading, time management, communications, study habits, or career selection. Can you think of others? Which methods will be most advantageous to you? Do you grasp things more easily through visual means, such as videos and books, or are you a listener who learns better with audio tapes? Do you need to interact with a live instructor? If you are a student, what grade-point average do you want to maintain?

Think also about rest and relaxation. Your mind needs this as well as your body. What techniques will serve you best (exercise, meditation, vacations, sleep, etc.)? How often will you use them and when?

After consideration of these issues, begin to write down your needs and your desires pertaining to this area. Then streamline your notes into specific goals.

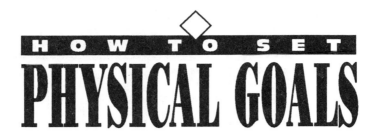

HOW TO SET
PHYSICAL GOALS

This one is pretty self-explanatory. What do you want to look like? More importantly, how concerned are you about keeping your body healthy and in good shape? How do you want to look to others?

PREPARATION CHECKLIST

1. Have paper and pen.
2. Be ready to think ...

THE GAME PLAN

In your quiet place, begin to think about your physical self. What things would you like to change? Which ones would you like to maintain as they are? Are you happy with your weight? How about your physical stamina? Are you healthy? Do you need more exercise? What types of sports and physical exercise do you participate in?

How about your image? What is your taste in fashion, and are you able to indulge that taste on your budget? How about your hair and makeup? (In our business, we have all the opportunities we need to experiment in this area!)

Also consider physical things outside of yourself that affect you. Are you living in the type of home, the area, the neighborhood, the type of terrain or climate you desire? Can you think of more questions to ask yourself pertaining to this area?

After you've answered these questions, make a list of things you want to change (mismanagement of time, over-eating, nervousness, worrying, chronic ailments, migraine headaches, smoking). Then list the positive things that already exist in your life and those you want to adopt (thinking ahead, patience, consideration of others). This is your outline for your goal list!

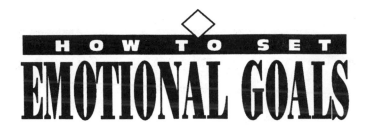

HOW TO SET EMOTIONAL GOALS

This area is very similar to the area of mental goals, but take your thought process out of your head and put it into your heart.

PREPARATION CHECKLIST

1. Have paper and pen.
2. Be ready to think...

THE GAME PLAN

Do you need to change any aspect of your emotional being? What must you do to achieve the following: love, peace of mind (and heart), relaxation, habit control, security, success, contentment, happiness, harmony (with yourself and with others), balance, quality of life, direction, and stability? Some people think emotions are thrust upon them, that they "can't help" the way they feel. This is not true. You can change the way you feel and react to things. It just takes a will and a plan.

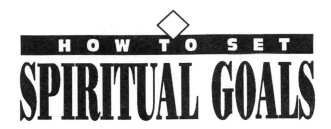

HOW TO SET SPIRITUAL GOALS

This area goes one step past emotions. Spirituality deals with your attitude toward life and everything in it, your belief in yourself, and something more.

PREPARATION CHECKLIST

1. Have paper and pen.
2. Be ready to think...

THE GAME PLAN

What can you do to become a more positive person? What do you want from life beyond the tangible, material rewards? What will you do to expand your beliefs and intuition this year? When will you begin, and how often will you work on these aspects of your life? Do you have peace of mind? These are things to think about when defining goals in this area.

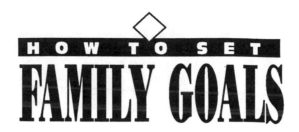

HOW TO SET FAMILY GOALS

This is the time to consider how you relate to those closest to you. Your family is your family, no matter how you feel about them — good or bad. Will you make changes here?

PREPARATION CHECKLIST

1. Have paper and pen.
2. Be ready to think...

THE GAME PLAN

What do you want in the part of your life that you share with your family — in the areas of love, respect, and closeness? What is the quality and quantity of the time you spend sharing activities together? How do you communicate with them? How do you express your feelings? If you're newly married, perhaps this is the year you want to start a family of your own. How big do you want your family to be in twenty years? Think about the adjustments you will have to make to accommodate your family's educational needs, cultural experiences, health needs, time demands, religious/spiritual fulfillments, vacations, and more. Obviously, when setting these goals, you will be influenced by and need to consider the feelings of others.

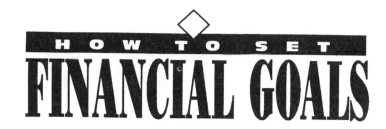

HOW TO SET FINANCIAL GOALS

Here's the area that probably causes more trouble for more people than any other, but you can master this aspect of your life by setting reachable goals.

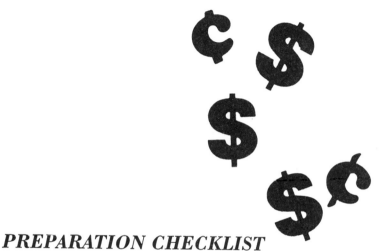

PREPARATION CHECKLIST

1. Have paper and pen.
2. Be ready to think...

THE GAME PLAN

What kind of income do you need to live at the standard to which you'd like to become accustomed? In other words, how much money do you need to be comfortable with your way of life? Consider the following financial demands: food, mortgage or rent payments, clothing, car, other transportation, insurances (health, auto, life, home, and disability), retirement fund, utilities, educational costs, taxes, child care, household products, household help, hair care, entertainment, newspapers, magazines, gifts, charitable contributions, vacations, legal fees, accounting fees, financial consulting. When you look at it, life can be really expensive! With good planning and solid goals, you can be on top of it.

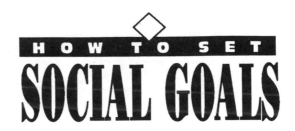

HOW TO SET
SOCIAL GOALS

Your social life is more than how many dates you've had this month or how often you and your spouse go out to dinner. It encompasses everything you do with other people outside of work, other than with your family. That's a pretty big chunk of your time. You can improve it if you're unhappy with it — and even if you're satisfied, it can get better with a plan!

PREPARATION CHECKLIST

1. List what you do now.
2. List what you want to do.
3. List what you would like to change.

THE GAME PLAN

In what types of sports, musical and cultural activities, and/or hobbies do you wish to participate? Who are your friends? Do you have a lot of casual acquaintances with whom you have "good times," or are you close to just one or two people? What type of person do you look for when seeking friendship? What type of character, behavior, values, interests? Do you prefer male or female friends? Does a person's age matter? How much influence do you think friends should have on each other?

How about other aspects of society? Do you want to be involved in community service — political, charitable, religious? And what kind of vacations would you like to take? Do you prefer a couple of days off here and there to break the routine, or do you want to be gone for a month at a time? Do you want relaxation, adventure, romance? And who do you want to take with you — some friends, your mate, the kids?

And finally, relating back to financial goals, how much do you want to spend on social activities? Every individual is unique, and you will come up with additional considerations in this area. Think it through. Decide what you want out of your social life, then set some goals and go after them!

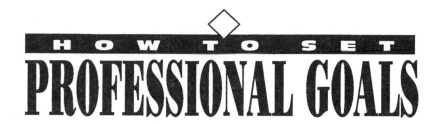

HOW TO SET
PROFESSIONAL GOALS

Many people define themselves by their professions. "Hi, I'm Geri. I'm a professional hair designer." Generally, your profession is your livelihood, the place where you spend most of your waking hours. A person ought to like his or her work, and, like anything, a profession is what you make it.

PREPARATION CHECKLIST

1. Have paper and pen.
2. Be ready to think...

THE GAME PLAN

Consider everything about your profession. What kind of industry, position, hours, income, challenges, freedom, creativity, people contact, benefits (health insurance, child care, and retirement programs, etc.) do you want? How much stimulation? What kind of a sense of fulfillment? Do you want it to be technical or non-technical? What about your employer — what kind of character, values, organizational skills, or culture do you want him or her to have? Where do you want to work? Do you anticipate joining any professional guilds, clubs, or associations? Do you wish to help others in your profession or to enhance your image or your organization's image?

Do you want to write about or teach your profession to others? If writing is an option, would you want your work to be published? Are you looking for awards or special recognition — some type of security (tangible or intangible)? How about specific guidance or additional instruction such as public speaking, management training, sales, planning skills, communications, or customer service? Perhaps classes in time management, writing skills, stress management, assertiveness, or psychology? Are you good at negotiations, crisis resolution, or decision making? Are you sensitive to others? These are all topics to think about when defining your professional goals.

The key to goal-setting is simple. Think about what you want out of life, and define it in some credible way. The key to making your goals a reality is BELIEVING IN YOURSELF.

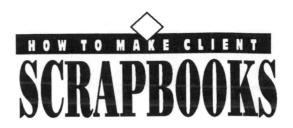

HOW TO MAKE CLIENT
SCRAPBOOKS

A scrapbook is not just a good way of keeping track of memories. It can be an excellent career tool, when used for makeovers, perm styles, colors, cuts, etc.— a way of showing clients your work or their own beauty potential.

PREPARATION CHECKLIST

Depending upon the type of book you are putting together, you will need some of the following items:

1. A three-ring binder.
2. Plastic page covers.
3. Identification tape with which to label your pictures.
4. A Polaroid camera for "before and after" pictures.
5. A bulletin board.

THE GAME PLAN

Each collection will have its own unique qualities. If you are doing a perm or color scrapbook, begin by cutting out pictures from magazines of the looks that interest you. Be sure to look for different textures, lengths, etc. Look also for different face shapes and what looks good on each one. You might even want to show some less attractive styles for the sake of contrast. Deal with specifics, such as different shapes of noses; high and low foreheads; or close or wide-set eyes. Show how to "balance" hairstyles and makeup. Demonstrate how to highlight positive features, play down negative ones, and correct perceived flaws.

If you are doing a "makeover" scrapbook, take "before" and "after" Polaroid shots of your models, pointing out the improvements you have made.

These scrapbooks are great to take along when you speak at seminars for women's groups or give special demonstrations. It's a convenient way of exhibiting your best accomplishments.

TIPS

- *Occasionally, you may want to take some of the "before and after" Polaroids out of your scrapbook and display them on a "brag board" in your shop so all of your customers can see your work.*
- *BE PROUD OF YOUR ACCOMPLISHMENTS, AND DON'T BE INHIBITED ABOUT DISPLAYING THEM. SUCCESS BEGINS WITH BELIEVING IN YOURSELF!*

MARKETING PROMOTIONS

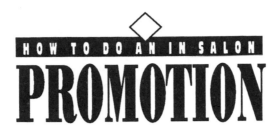

HOW TO DO AN IN SALON
PROMOTION

Promotions are great business. They can cause excitement among existing clients, while bringing in new ones.

PREPARATION CHECKLIST

Get a pencil and paper (or a secretary) and decide what your promotion will be.

THE GAME PLAN

When you have an idea in mind, begin by breaking it down. What will it cost? How much will you spend on the giveaway? How much will you give designers for their participation? What will you give to the winner of the contest? For example, you may choose to give a trip. What is the expense? How long will it be? Then put the whole package together, check with a travel agency, and find out the exact cost prior to doing the promotion.

How are you going to advertise, and what kinds of banners or flyers will you need to let clients know about it? Will it be just for regular clients or advertised through outside sales or newspapers and magazines? How long will it last?

Set the rules and regulations of any contests. Plan contests at least three months ahead of time so that you are able to do everything and have everything made. Decide on all of the features and benefits of the contest to the salon. List all the pros and cons, and plan for the worst-case scenario to make sure expenses could still be covered; then have a staff meeting to inform your people what you're planning and get their input. Without their consent and participation, you could have a mess on your hands. Excite them about the idea, and reward them with something that will be exciting to them. Staff prizes could be educational classes, bonuses, time off, or something that has meaning to an individual.

The planning stages of your promo are most important. All of the preparations must be thoroughly thought out and prioritized. It's important to know that everything is ready to go at least a couple of weeks ahead of time so people are aware of what is happening. Hang your banners and give out materials in enough time so people can get prepared for the event. At the actual time of the promo, follow up and keep your staff updated about what is happening on a daily or weekly basis. Continuously encourage your people. Without a good attitude on the part of your staff, any promotion could be a flop. Keep them motivated. When it's over, make sure there is no cheating or bending the rules for anyone.

Some "promo pros": Promos cause excitement in the salon, an opportunity for clients to win something, and an opportunity for the staff to get something back for their work. They can encourage more sales; you should be able to generate more income with a promo. They should always lead to more sales.

The cons: Maybe your staff doesn't like the idea, therefore they do nothing, and it could cost you money. If you've never done it before, you can't be sure it will be a success. It's very important to monitor how the promotion is working, and to write a report at the end to gauge whether or not it should be done again. This report should account for financial aspects, so you know how much the promotion costs and what you made. Then you decide if it was worth the time and effort. Of course, you keep records so you can refer back to them.

TIPS

- *When choosing a bonus for your staff, be sure to make it something everyone will want. If it is a personal gift, for example, don't give a pair of shears to someone who already has two or three pairs.*
- *If you choose an "open" educational, be sure to put a limit on the potential cost and the time during which it can be taken.*
- *USE YOUR IMAGINATION. THE REWARDS ARE WORTH A LITTLE THOUGHT!*

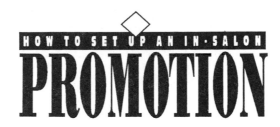

HOW TO SET UP AN IN·SALON PROMOTION

An in-salon promotion can be very successful in promoting a product or service to your existing clients. This is a great way to give something back to clients who are always there week after week or month after month. Of course, any new client can take advantage of the special offer as well.

PREPARATION CHECKLIST

Before you initiate your promo, have a storyboarding session. Decide the following:
1. What do you want to do?
2. How much do you want to spend?
3. What supplies do you need to buy?
4. How will you administer it?

THE GAME PLAN

Have some large posters or signs made. Make sure they are tastefully done. Frame them if possible, and display them in the reception area or the entrance, in the dressing rooms, bathrooms, and at the stations or on the mirrors. Make up some banners to hang from the ceiling and some buttons for your staff to wear saying, "Ask me about our special promo." It's a good incentive for your staff to offer a bonus for the employee who sells the most promo specials. If that is not an option, make sure that you recognize the top performer in some way.

Be sure to have all of your products ordered well in advance and in stock before the promotion. Also, don't forget to inform all of your receptionists about the special so that they can be selling and suggesting it over the telephone when clients call in for appointments. Monitor the services and retail products being sold, all expenses incurred, and all revenue coming in through the special.

Finally, keep a file containing all of your promo information: how it was done, the costs involved, the features and benefits, whether or not it was profitable, and ideas and suggestions about how to improve it next time. Also include the names and telephone numbers of all of the vendors used for banners, pins, products, etc.

TIPS

- *Give yourself at least two months to prepare for a promo. This will give you ample time to order your products, advertising visuals, etc. Throwing things together can cause a lot of stress and cost a lot of money.*
- *SPECIALS CAN BE FUN AND BRING IN A LOT OF MONEY. GO FOR IT!*

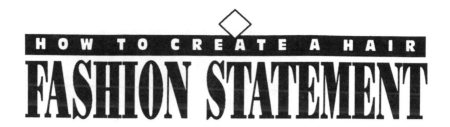

HOW TO CREATE A HAIR
FASHION STATEMENT

Doing a photo session gives your staff great motivation, and creating a fashion statement for your salon is a fantastic way of getting everyone involved in a project together. It also encourages them to find out what's happening in fashion and teaches them how to look for models as well as promoting awareness of what's going on in the industry for that season.

PREPARATION CHECKLIST

1. Gather as many good fashion magazines as you can get your hands on. Look especially for European magazines such as *Vogue* of London, Paris, Rome, as well as others.
2. Look for a good photographer modeling agency.

THE GAME PLAN

When planning a hair fashion statement, do it for the upcoming season — fall/winter or spring/summer. Begin by having a meeting where you discuss all the possibilities — the newest looks that you may encounter. Look through all of the magazines you've gathered and discover what's happening in fashion. Fashion will dictate what's happening in hair. You will notice, as you go through the European magazines, that London is strong on hair, while Italy spotlights clothing, and France's forte is design.

Find the look that you think is going to "happen" and work six months ahead. Then put your fashion statement together. Look for textures, colors, and style (clothing). Observe the hairstyles. Are they sleek, full, or rounded? Square, short, or long? You'll find all of the information you need in these magazines.

Once your statement is established, your next step is to decide what types of models, haircuts, and styles you want to present. Have your models come in, and bring the outfits you plan for them to wear. Having them collectively try them on will help you see if you've achieved a single theme or idea. It is important that your photographs project a collection — that they follow a theme — that the clothing or backdrops or backgrounds are coordinated. You want it to look like a group photo session rather than several individual photos. Your next step is to find a photographer. Make sure that he or she understands what you are trying to accomplish. (Refer to the questions in the chapter titled "How to Interview a Photographer.")

This project can be a lot of fun, as well as stirring up the imagination and creativity of your staff. It will give them a feeling of teamwork, togetherness, and excitement once the photography is all done and published and clients come back and say, "I saw your name, salon, or work in a magazine!"

TIPS

- *Make sure your whole staff is included in this project. It can be a great boon to those who are shy or less sure of themselves. (And they may surprise you!)*
- *YOUR SALON CAN BE A FASHION MAKER INSTEAD OF A FASHION FOLLOWER!*

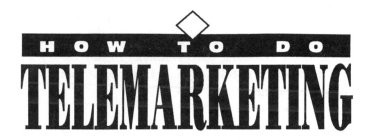

HOW TO DO
TELEMARKETING

Telemarketing is a means of promoting inside your salon or hiring an outside person to do telephone soliciting for you. It's a great tool to attract business and gauge the business you have.

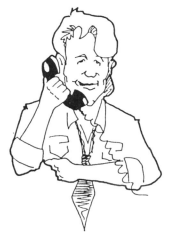

PREPARATION CHECKLIST

To prepare for this, you will need to have in mind the kind of information you require and to have a complete list of the customers you want to contact. It's best if your telephone list is computerized.

THE GAME PLAN

You can use telephone marketing in your salon any time someone is available to spend time talking on the phone to your clients. This type of advertising has many distinct advantages. It's a personal approach. You're communicating directly with your client one to one. You are also getting the response immediately. When you send out surveys, customers may not mail them back right away (or at all), but they are usually willing to answer questions on the phone.

Plan ahead. Know what you'd like to accomplish. When telemarketing, you may want to ask a new client how the service was, how the work was, and if he or she would return to the salon. You may ask if he or she has any questions or comments about the first visit. All of this could be done very easily by the front desk person or a staff member who doesn't have anything to do for awhile.

If you're trying to mass market your salon, it will be more beneficial to hire an outside telemarketing company. It will be your responsibility to tell them what you're promoting and to come up with a script for them to use. You may want to do a survey on why customers have not returned to your salon, what clients' needs might be, or whether the services are satisfactory.

Cost for this service varies greatly. Call your local marketing survey companies to get quotes, and shop around. It could save you money. Also, make sure that the company you hire uses professional telemarketers to do the job.

You can hire telemarketing people for any time frame. You might want to try it for a month, two months, or just a week or so.

Telemarketing can be very beneficial, but you need computerized telephone lists in order to do it. If you don't have good records, compiling telephone numbers can be extremely time-consuming and hardly worth the effort. Make sure you have a complete list of your clients and their telephone numbers. If you are looking for new customers, you can try buying telephone lists. The company you contact can tell you where to buy them. They are usually categorized according to lifestyle, income, or geographical area. This helps you pinpoint the type of clientele that interests you. Make sure you market to people who would fit in with your type of salon. Don't market to high-end people if you are a low-end salon. It's important to know what your marketing tactics are.

TIPS

- *When hiring an outside telemarketing firm, you might want to ask them to call you back with their "pitch." This will tell you exactly what they are going to say and how it will sound to your customers.*
- *USE THIS TACTIC TO GATHER ALMOST ANY KIND OF CLIENT INFORMATION YOU NEED!*

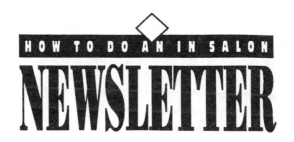

HOW TO DO AN IN SALON
NEWSLETTER

An in-salon newsletter is probably one of the best ways to communicate with your clients. It's also a great way to promote your designers, your products, and your services. Make it as elaborate or as simple as you like, but make it interesting and informative.

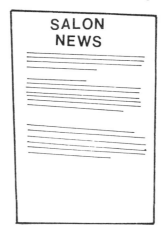

PREPARATION CHECKLIST

1. Decide how often to publish your newsletter. Suggestions: Twice a year, "Spring and Summer" and "Fall and Winter," or four times a year, one for each season.
2. Choose someone to collect information about everything that anyone in your shop is involved in: shows, photo sessions, cut-a-thons, charity events, awards, contests, etc. Also collect all the latest info on what's hot in hair and fashion.
3. Find someone (among your staff or outside) who can put all the information into newsletter form. Keep it short and simple.
4. Decide on the format and the logo you want to use. (What color paper, ink; what kind and size of print.)
5. Get estimates on printing prices.

THE GAME PLAN

Once you've collected everyone's ideas and gathered your data, the rest is up to your writer. Work with him or her in the beginning to make sure you get exactly what you have in mind.

118

The following is a list of suggested topics that you might want to include in your newsletter:

- *The latest hair trends.*
- *The up-and-coming clothing looks, colors, and styles.*
- *What's happening in your salon.*
- *What new and exciting things you and your designers are doing.*
- *Current and upcoming specials or promotions on products and services.*
- *Tips on hair, skin, makeup, bodycare, and fitness.*
- *Special recipes for a healthier you.*
- *Articles on clients who may be in the limelight.*
- *Makeovers — before and after pictures of your clients.*

TIPS

- *Make up some coupons for your newsletter for products or services. This will give you some idea of who is reading it!*
- *Get creative with your artwork. Use a staff member with a flair for drawing, or get a book of "clip art" (available in any stationery or office supply store).*
- *Grab your reader's attention, then keep it short and to the point.*
- *Give yourself (or your writer) enough time. For example, a fall-winter release must be started in June or July.*
- *Use photos from your own shoots. This is an opportunity to show off your work!*
- *Use your salon logo or get a new one just for your newsletter.*
- *Make sure you have your salon name, address, and phone number on the newsletter. If you are going to mail it out, leave one side blank for clients' names and addresses.*
- *HAVE FUN WITH THIS PROJECT!*

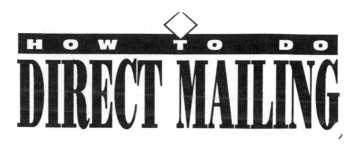

DIRECT MAILING

Direct mailing is probably the most advantageous of all types of advertising and marketing for you to do, especially if you mail to your existing clientele. They know and like you and are more likely to purchase what you are offering.

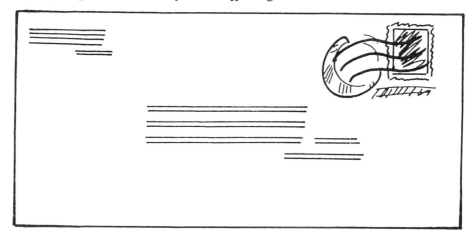

PREPARATION CHECKLIST

1. Call mailing houses to get rates.
2. Talk to people who have experience in direct mailing.

THE GAME PLAN

To begin with, it is important that you design what you are trying to present in a very fashionable manner. If it is a special on permanent waves or color, have a nice picture or sketch on the back of your postcard or flyer. You will probably find that it is more cost effective to use a postcard rather than enclose your piece in an envelope; however, for a more formal or personal special, use an envelope.

In order to effectively use direct mail in your salon, it is almost imperative that you own a computer. It's really too time-consuming to go through all of your customer files and copy each one individually; it's much easier to have your computer print out labels. It is also extremely important to keep track of people who respond to mailings. Your computer can do this with codes; otherwise, have the clients bring in their postcards when they come in for the service you are offering. If you don't know your rate of return, your mailing won't do you any good. Your return will tell you if it was worth doing and if you should do it again, or if you should try something else next time.

It's important to plan ahead. Having something typeset and printed takes time. You must allow for possible mistakes. Be sure to give yourself enough time to prepare and get your postcards written out so that you are not sending them too close to the time of the promo. Plan to begin at least a couple of months before the promotion is scheduled to begin so you can work at an easier pace and not have to race around at the last minute.

TIPS

- *It is extremely important to keep your files updated. Your computer can help here. It can tell you if a client has been in recently or perhaps has moved away. This will save on postage because you will not be sending pieces to former clients who are no longer available.*
- *IF ONE TYPE OF MAILING DOESN'T WORK FOR YOU, TRY SOMETHING ELSE. GET CREATIVE. IT'S WHAT THIS BUSINESS IS ALL ABOUT!*

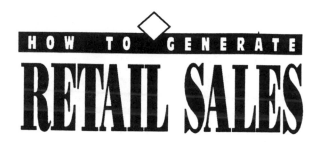

HOW TO GENERATE
RETAIL SALES

Fine department stores are doing it! Neighborhood drugstores are doing it! YOUR COMPETITION IS DOING IT!! There is no doubt about it. Retailing is here to stay. Whether you choose to sell fine brand names or you bring out a line of products all your own, retailing is important to your business!

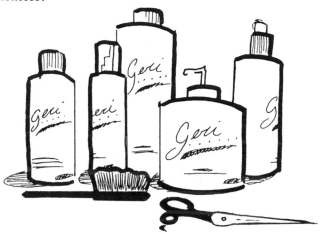

PREPARATION CHECKLIST

Long before you order your first supply of products, you will need to consider the following:
1. Sales training classes for staff and owner.
2. Product knowledge.
3. Choice of goods to purchase.
4. Ordering procedures.
5. Inventory information.
6. Freight and shipping information.
7. Opening accounts with vendors.
8. Terms of payment.
9. Product turnover.
10. Stocking inventory.
11. Display techniques, including design and lighting.
12. Where to purchase shelving and display cases.
13. Controlling product loss.
14. Computerizing front desk for inventory control.

15. Compensation for staff sales.
16. Sales goals for staff.
17. Incentive and bonus packages.
18. How to set up and organize contests

THE GAME PLAN

The most important thing is to learn how to sell. Large corporations are continually training their people in sales. Your objective is the same. Why not follow their lead? There are sales seminars available, such as Dale Carnegie, Career Track, and Earl Nightingale Co., that can teach your staff to become sales oriented. Many colleges and high schools have courses available, and you can even look into "do it yourself" courses with audio and video tapes.

TIPS

- *Invite speakers from the business world to come and talk to your staff. They can be a great choice for your staff meetings. (See "How to Conduct a Staff Meeting.") Have them talk about several subjects, from "Customer Service" and "Personalities" to "Handling Problem Clients" and "Closing a Sale."*
- *Make sure your designers are familiar with the products you are selling so they can recommend them intelligently.*
- *Consider your clientele when deciding on a product line. Choose products that will appeal to most of your consumers.*
- *REMEMBER, EDUCATION IS THE KEY TO A MILLION DOLLAR BUSINESS!*

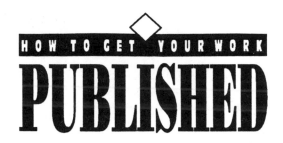

HOW TO GET YOUR WORK
PUBLISHED

There is nothing more rewarding to a hairstylist or makeup artist than having work published in a magazine. And so many magazines are looking for good photographs and articles, all you need to do is to supply them with the information and pictures. Here are a few things you should know before you begin.

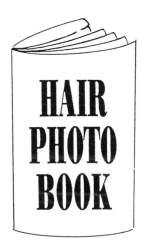

PREPARATION CHECKLIST

1. Make sure all of the information you have is current, newsworthy, and informative to their readers.
2. Make sure your photos are top-quality prints — 8" x 10" prints or color transparencies are preferred.
3. Make sure all hairstyles and makeup are up-to-date or ahead of their time, because it takes at least three to six months before anything can get printed.
4. Make sure that you send the right kinds of pictures to the right magazines. If you are sending an artistic hair fashion look to a commercial magazine, they will not print it. You need to meet their requirements. If you have any doubts, call and ask the editor.
5. Know the deadlines for the magazines in which you are interested.
6. Make sure you are working on the season ahead.

THE GAME PLAN

Find the magazines that interest you by looking on newsstands and at hair shows. Get their addresses and write to them requesting deadlines, what looks they need, on what season they are working, and what information they would like to have. Do a photo session especially for those magazines. Use a professional photographer, because portrait photos are difficult, and use a model with a great face. Get one good original shot and have a local printer reproduce it for you. Get as many prints as you will need, and have the printer put your credits right on the photo. These should include your logo, the hairdresser, the makeup artist, the photographer, the clothing designer or shop that supplied the fashions, the photo stylist, and anyone else who you feel should get credit. Make sure you get a release form from the photographer and model or agency for your uses.

Write a brief description of the hairstyle and how you achieved the look, and have a professional press release folder accompany your photos or articles. Enclose a cover letter with all of your information, asking them to review your work. Send everything by registered mail or return requested so you know that it has been received, and make sure you address it to the proper person. This is even more important if you are sending materials overseas.

Now just wait a few months and see!

TIPS

- *Many magazines will send you copies of the issues in which they use your work. Be sure to ask.*
- *DON'T BE INTIMIDATED. IT'S NOT THAT HARD TO GET PUBLISHED.*

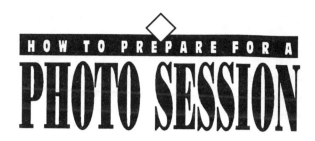

HOW TO PREPARE FOR A
PHOTO SESSION

*For resumes, for advertising purposes, to get your work published, even for staff morale —
it is helpful to show people your creations. And there is no better way than to have them
photographed.*

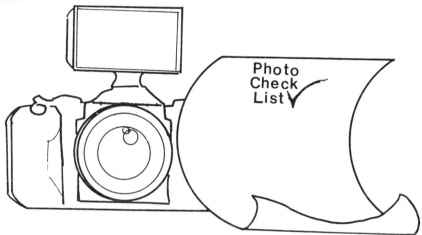

Photo
Check
List ✓

PREPARATION CHECKLIST

1. Set up a meeting with your staff specifically to discuss a photography session. Have
   them bring ideas for great new looks from magazines (*Vogue, Elle, Taxi...*), European books, newspaper clippings, hairstyle books, etc.
2. Be ready with all of the tools needed to do a storyboard.
3. Make a list of professional photographers whose work and reputation you respect
   and admire.

THE GAME PLAN

At your staff meeting, look at the pictures your people bring in. This is the time for
enthusiasm to be high. Get everyone's opinions and suggestions and discuss them. Write
everything down for future reference.

Next, storyboard all ideas. Some suggestions are:

1. Season; 2. Mood; 3. Feeling; 4. Style; 5. Clothes; 6. Jewelry; 7. Location shot; 8. Models;
9. Backdrop; 10. Props; 11. Makeup; 12. Art stylist — props; 13. Photo stylist — clothes,
accessories; 14. Time frame; 15. Photographer; 16. Photo application usage; 17. Dates open;
18. Hair designer; and 19. Budget.

Finally, make some appointments with photographers. Interview them. Check out their work and look at their portfolios. Make sure you choose a photographer who has done fashion, hair, etc. Now you're ready!

TIPS

- *Don't discount anyone's thoughts or opinions without first discussing them with everyone. Sometimes the best ideas come out of left field!*
- *Always focus on the season to come. If it is spring or summer, concentrate on fall/winter. Conversely, if it is fall or winter, concentrate on spring/summer.*
- *REMEMBER, PHOTOGRAPHS LAST. CHOOSE A GREAT MODEL AND PRESENT YOUR VERY BEST WORK!*

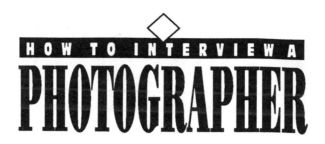

HOW TO INTERVIEW A
PHOTOGRAPHER

Selecting your photographer is vital to having the very best results. You need someone who has experience in fashion photography and whose work pleases you, but it is equally important to choose someone who you can trust. If you are just beginning or looking for someone new, then the interview process is crucial for making the right choice.

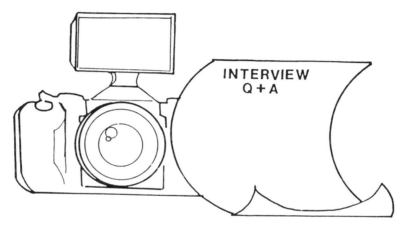

INTERVIEW
Q + A

PREPARATION CHECKLIST

Have the following things ready to bring with you when you interview your photographer:
1. Storyboard from staff.
2. Pictures of moods, feelings, style, backgrounds, etc. on which you have decided.
3. Pictures that show the clarity of color or black/white and high/low contrast in which you are interested.
4. A list of applications or usage:
   A. Kind of film you want for pictures.
   B. Slides — what size? — B/W or color?
   C. Prints — B/W or color?
       i. On what kind of paper do you want them printed?
       ii. Glossy or flat finish?
   D. Reproduction use:
       i. Magazines
       ii. Newspapers

      iii. Brochures
      iv. Stationery cards
      v. Billboards
      vi. Wall art
      vii. Posters
      viii. Videos
      ix. Slide shows

    E. A checklist of your wants and needs to give to the photographer. (A safety cover for you.)

THE GAME PLAN

An interview is a question-and-answer session during which you (hopefully) receive information from the photographer. Here are some suggestions.:

1. Ask to see a portfolio of all hair and fashion work he or she has done.
2. Has he or she done any fashion work for magazines, newspapers, videos, etc.? (Ask to see tear sheets or brochures.)
3. Ask for references from modeling agencies, magazines, modeling schools, newspapers, department stores, catalogs, etc.
4. Does the photographer work on location or have a studio?
5. Does he or she have an assistant, makeup artist, or photo stylist?
6. Ask about the price of services — hourly rate, half-day rate, full-day rate. What services do you get for the price? Are the prices of film and supplies included?
7. What kind of equipment is used? (Camera sizes, lights, background props, etc.)
8. If assistants are used, is there an extra charge?
9. Do you pay expenses for location shots, or are they included in the day rate?
10. How long will it take to receive finished products?
11. Are you expected to pay before or after the shoot?
12. Can the photographer supply models? Price per hour? Day?
13. Does he or she shoot Polaroids first?

TIPS

- *Ask friends in the business for their recommendations when you first start looking for a good photographer.*
- *TRUST YOUR INSTINCTS, AND HAVE A GREAT SESSION!*

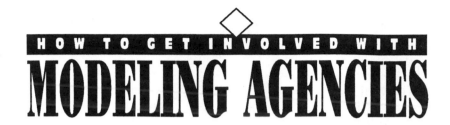

MODELING AGENCIES

Having contacts with modeling and casting agencies can be beneficial for your business and for you personally. You will have better access to models you might need for your photo sessions, and it can help to drum up new business with people you enjoy working on, who will generally allow you to be very creative.

PREPARATION CHECKLIST

Make a list of any agencies in your area. Then gather together your bio, any press releases, photos of your work, and anything for which you have been given credit that you feel would be interesting to them.

THE GAME PLAN

The first thing to do is contact the agencies on your list. Send them a bio and the other information you have collected. When talking to them, make sure that you are specific about your objectives. Ask if you can do hair for them at a photo session. Offer discount services in your salon to the models. Ask for an appointment to discuss some of these possibilities. Try to come up with a suitable price structure that will give the models a discount while still leaving you a reasonable profit. Offer to do educational classes for them on how to take care of their hair or makeup or how to take care of themselves when out on a shoot — what to bring with them, how to do hair different ways, and what products to use.

Assure the agency that you won't be overly creative. Sometimes models have jobs that they were hired for based on the length of their hair or for their specific appearance. Ask the agency for recommendations on how they want their girls to look. You might suggest a bartering deal to your models — if you cut their hair, they will do a sitting for you for a photo session or you will get a discount on their hourly rate. Find out if you can use them in a fashion show. Always agree not to use the photos for anything other than promotions. Be aware that if there is money involved, both the model and the agency get their cut.

When working with theater people, you may be able to be more creative, but remember, they may need specific looks for certain roles, and you need to be willing and able to accommodate them.

TIPS

- *Develop a good rapport with the models or actors. Don't treat them (or anyone, for that matter) as though you are superior to them. Listen to them when doing their hair or makeup, as you would with any client.*
- *Try to think of other creative ways to trade your expertise for a model's or an actor's services.*
- *THESE ARE THE PEOPLE WITH WHOM YOU CAN TAKE THE "EVERYDAY" OUT OF YOUR JOB. HAVE FUN WITH THEM!*

microdembrasion

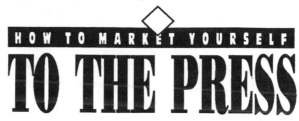

HOW TO MARKET YOURSELF
TO THE PRESS

When you market yourself to the press, you want to present the most positive impression possible. You are using this vehicle to sell yourself, so you want to present yourself in the most flattering light.

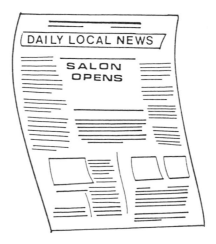

PREPARATION CHECKLIST

You will need to put together a bio (See "How to Prepare a Personal Bio") and have a flattering, professional photograph taken.

THE GAME PLAN

To do this properly, you must take the time to put together a press kit, including your bio and picture. Place it all in a nice folder with your logo, some salon stationery for letters, and your business cards. Each time you have done something newsworthy or you have an idea about which they might be interested in writing, put your press kit together. Make it brief, easy to read, and easy to understand. If it is too long, they won't look at it. Make sure it is neat, typed clearly, and that there is a good ribbon in your typewriter or computer. Use professional looking stationery. Place your photo and bio in one pocket and the information on the opposite side with your business card. Don't hesitate to send anything you feel might interest them. The more information you send to the press, the more likely they are to pick up a story.

TIPS

- *When you have a photograph taken, make sure that the likeness is flattering, but looks professional. This is not the time to have a "romantic" or "bizarre" look unless that is your trademark.*
- *Most likely, the press will not print the first article you send to them, nor perhaps many of the things that you send, but the more that they hear from you, the more likely they are to remember your name when they need something written on the newest looks in hair length or some other topic concerning hair fashion.*
- *BELIEVE IN YOURSELF, AND DON'T GET DISCOURAGED!*

HAIR OR MAKEUP IN THE MOVIES

The movie industry can be exciting, and people involved in it are always looking for free-lance hairdressers or makeup artists to fill in when someone can't be there. This is where you can get a start.

PREPARATION CHECKLIST

Check your city's chamber of commerce to see if any movies will be shot in the area. (If you are very serious about this type of career, you may have to consider relocating to Los Angeles, New York, certain cities in Florida, or even Pittsburgh, Pennsylvania, where a lot of films have been shot in the last few years.) Ask them for locations and film directories.

THE GAME PLAN

The film directory you receive should list the names of agents who hire all the makeup artists and hairdressers for movies. Call casting companies and see if you can send a resume. Ask them for any information they can give that will help you get a start in the movie industry. Find out how you can have your name put on a list from which they might choose designers and/or makeup artists.

Your resume is very important. It's helpful if you have experience in special effects such as hairpieces, wigs, toupees, or any kind of add-on hair. You also need to have very good styling abilities and be quick. If you're interested in makeup, highlight your experience in latex application or other theatrical looks. Generally makeup and hair people are separate.

If you do one, you usually don't do the other unless it's a low-budget film, so be specific about what your strong points are. After you've done the leg work, ask if you can come and observe.

Some of the pros and cons of this type of work: You can be tied up for weeks or months at a time. This interferes with a steady job. The hours are long — sometimes fourteen hours, beginning at 4 or 5 A.M. If you're interested in part-time work, specify on your application how much time you have available. Consider being an assistant so your hours are less rigorous. It's a lot of hard work all at once, with long waits while they shoot. Most of the hairdressers who work on main actors are there for the duration of the picture, working six days a week. You work in all kinds of weather conditions. Call time can be any time, and there can be lots of schedule changes. Nothing is ever organized, because you never know what will happen the day before. You must be flexible and adaptable. Depending on the budget, pay structure could be from $10 per hour to $2 – 3,000 per week.

Once you have worked on a film, your name is usually passed around to all of the other workers. If you do a good job, they may refer you to others.

TIPS

- *When contacting a casting company, be sure to get the name of the person you should contact.*
- *IF YOU'RE NOT READY FOR THE "BIG TIME" TRY DOING SOME COMMUNITY THEATER WORK. IT'S CREATIVE, AND GREAT EXPERIENCE.*

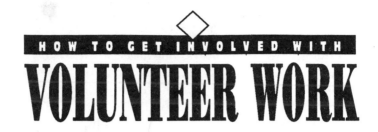

HOW TO GET INVOLVED WITH
VOLUNTEER WORK

Many associations and charities need and want someone to help them raise funds. This can be rewarding for you, both internally and externally. You have the opportunity for some excellent publicity and, more importantly, you can really help a lot of people.

PREPARATION CHECKLIST

List some possible charities or organizations with whom you would like to work. Then have a brainstorming session and decide what potential ideas you might want to use to raise money.

THE GAME PLAN

Once you know what you'd like to do (for example, run a cut-a-thon or a show), contact the charity that interests you. Ask if they would be interested in your idea or promotion. Make an appointment with the directors of the organization, and present your plan to them. Ask if they have anyone who can help. Get all of your information together, then gather a committee to promote the presentation. Find people who will help you market and advertise. Try to get someone to donate printing services, art work, decorating skills, food, space, and anything else you can think of that you will need. Look for people with the time to donate and who are willing to put in the effort.

Your budget is very important. Who is going to be responsible for collecting funds? Try to get the charity to help raise capital through its fund-raiser list.

If you are not putting the show together, you can volunteer your time and service as an individual. Many places, such as children's hospitals, old-age homes, or hospices, will welcome you with open arms. Contact these places. Sometimes people don't have visitors, and yours might be the only outside face they see, so it can be very rewarding. Other possibilities are shelters for the homeless or for battered women. Sometimes women are hiding from people who want to hurt them and are afraid to go out. Try reading to someone who is blind, or think of other things you can do.

TIPS

- *ASIDE FROM THE PUBLICITY, DON'T UNDERESTIMATE THE PERSONAL REWARDS YOU CAN RECEIVE FROM THIS KIND OF WORK!*